New Life

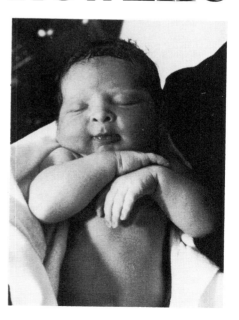

JANET & ARTHUR BALASKAS

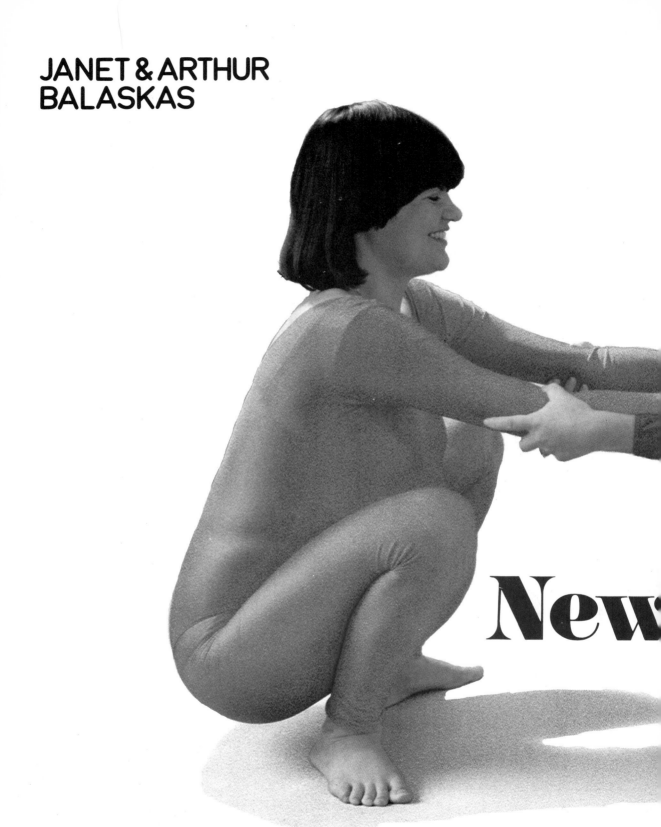

New

FOREWORD BY MICHEL ODENT

THE BOOK OF EXERCISES FOR CHILDBIRTH

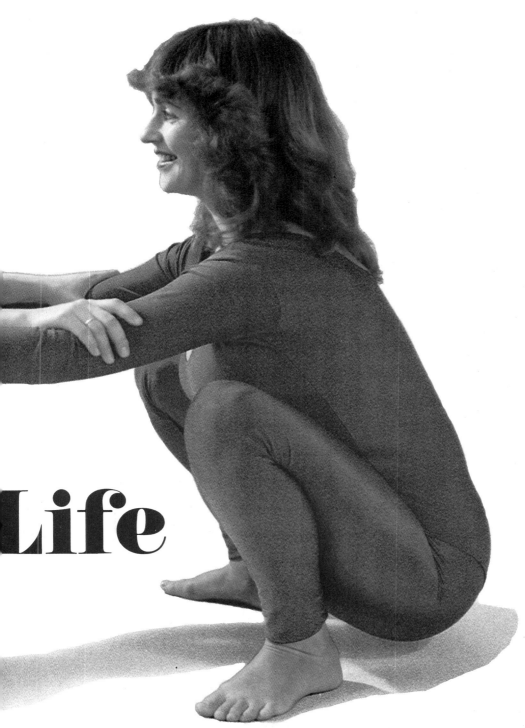

Life

SIDGWICK & JACKSON LONDON

To our daughters,
Kira, Nina, and Kim

Our sincere thanks to all the
families who have contributed to the
creation of this book, for all they
have taught us and for the use of
the photographs which illuminate
the text. The authors and publisher
would also like to thank Dorothee
von Greiff, who took the
photographs for the original edition
of *New Life*. They would also like to
thank Sandra Lusada and Conde
Nast Publications (*Vogue*,
November 1982) for the photograph
on pages 48–9, and Anthea
Sieveking and Vision International
for the photographs on the inside
front cover and the title page, and
on pages 41, 54, 55, 64–5, 71, 72,
78, 79, 84, 85, 89, 110, 117, 118 and
119.

For classes in the Balaskas
method of preparation for
Active Birth, contact:

The Active Birth Movement,
32 Willow Road,
London NW3
01-794 5227

First published in Great Britain by
Sidgwick and Jackson Limited in 1979

This revised edition first published in
Great Britain by Sidgwick and Jackson
Limited in 1983

Copyright © 1979 Arthur and Janet Balaskas

0-283-98997-1 (softcover)

Designed by Paul Watkins

Printed in Great Britain by Anchor Press
and bound by William Brendon
both of Tiptree, Essex
for Sidgwick and Jackson Limited
1 Tavistock Chambers, Bloomsbury Way
London WC1A 2SG

Contents

FOREWORD

My answer was unhesitatingly yes when Janet Balaskas asked
me to write a foreword to the new edition of *New Life*. As a
matter of fact, I am proud to introduce a book which is both so
simple and so important. It is exactly the book that Janet, with
the help of her husband Arthur, could write and had to write.

I don't want to say anything about the book itself. You'll look
at it, you'll read it, you'll study some chapters and you'll
meditate about some key paragraphs. You'll understand better
why this book is the one which can help you so much when you
know more about the author, whose personal qualities show
through many pages of the book. She is the kind of person we
have to listen to, and even to follow.

Janet is an enthusiastic person, which means, literally, or
etymologically, that she is guided by *theos* – by God. She is
endowed with a powerful and irresistible vital strength; she can
face most of the difficulties we have to cope with during a
lifetime; she is strong because she has convictions and she wants
to share them. She is convinced that one cannot change life
without changing childbirth first. This might be the meaning of
New Life. We need to meet enthusiastic people.

Janet is an ante-natal teacher. Women from other civilizations
might be astonished to discover that modern women need ante-
natal teachers. Why is it necessary in our society to teach
everything? Even how to give birth, how to breastfeed, and
how to make love? One might give many answers, but one of the
main explanations is certainly that some of our vital functions
are commonly disturbed in our civilization – our neuro-
endocrinological system is commonly out of order. In other
words, we are losing our instincts. It is as if the set point level
of our key hormone-regulating brain structures, namely the
'hypothalamo-limbic system', was commonly altered as early as
foetal life, birth and infancy, by pathogenic situations which
arise too frequently. So a delivery which is difficult, though for
no anatomical reason, may be considered as a disease of
civilization and a difficult birth is one of these pathogenic
situations which will directly or indirectly trigger other ones. It

is a vicious circle. The ante-natal teacher, by helping women to give birth with a minimal use of drugs and intervention, contributes to the breaking of this vicious circle.

Janet is also a mother. We must listen to mothers. They have a specific knowledge and understanding of life. Nowadays one is permitted to claim that our planet is in danger because it is ruled by male human beings: men control everything, even childbirth. The first stage in an effective global revolution might be when male doctors accept progressively to retire from obstetrics and give back childbirth to women.

Michel Odent

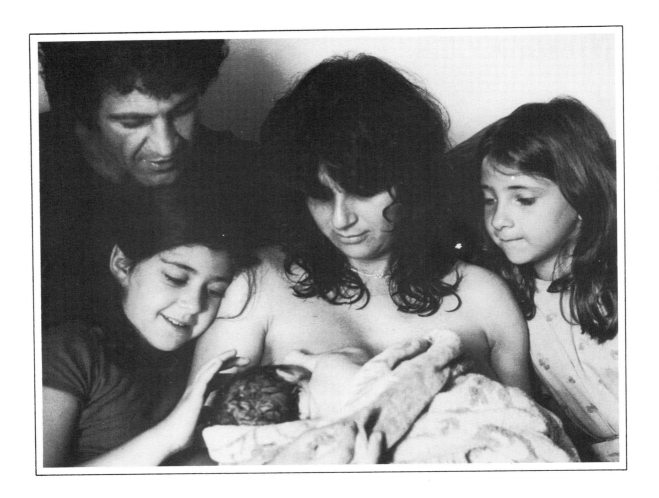

INTRODUCTION

I have given birth to three children.

I was 24 years old when I became pregnant with my daughter Nina. This was my first experience of birth and I prepared myself by reading all the popular books written on the subject and by attending ante-natal classes at the maternity home where she was born, in Johannesburg. I wanted a spontaneous birth and prepared myself to avoid taking drugs by learning to use my breathing as an aid for labour. Like many women I found this very helpful, and have 'breathed' my way through the births of all my children.

I also regularly practised the popular exercises derived from physiotherapy which were done lying down on the floor. They were relaxing and restful at the time but did nothing to fundamentally relax the tension in my body or to improve my postural sense. They also had the disadvantage of conditioning one to expect to lie down in labour.

On the day of the birth, I was advised to stay active in the early first stage, but as soon as the contractions became intense, I lay down in bed propped up by pillows, in a semi-sitting, reclining position and stayed like that throughout. I took no painkillers but was given a 'mild muscle relaxant' and later an episiotomy, despite my pleas to the contrary. I pushed Nina out in the semi-sitting position. The episiotomy made the 2nd stage fairly easy despite the fact that I was pushing 'uphill'. I felt uncomfortable and painful for weeks after the birth and it was months before my pelvic floor felt normal again.

Some years later I joined the National Childbirth Trust and became an ante-natal teacher, holding preparation classes for pregnant women and their partners in my home. I had been practising stretching exercises for a few years with my husband. We began to experiment with postures to find out which were suitable for childbirth; we concentrated mainly on those which increased the flexibility of the pelvic area and several of the mothers in my classes practised them throughout their pregnancies. All the women doing the exercises I suggested reported that they felt very relaxed and healthy and enjoyed the effects of the sessions.

When I became pregnant for the second time, I wanted Kim to be born at home. I practised the stretching exercises regularly. During her birth I was active in the early first stage and once again sat in bed when the contractions became strong. With all the preparation I had done I was surprised that the first stage was very long and was complaining to my friendly GP that I seemed to be stuck. He had recently returned from a working holiday in Botswana where he observed African women giving birth. He suggested that I should get up and do some squatting and make the most of the contractions. This was immediately helpful but I found it very difficult squatting with my slightly stiff, civilized ankles and ended up kneeling forward onto the bed until transition — when I reverted to the tried and familiar semi-sitting, reclining position. Kim was born without an episiotomy despite an unusually large head and weighed in at 8 lbs 4 oz. It certainly was an effort to push her out — and although I was lucky to escape a tear, my pelvic floor was grazed and tender and my lower back ached for several weeks after the birth.

Mulling over the birth with my husband and friends I realized what most primitive women in the world instinctively know, how important it is to keep moving and to adopt sensible positions throughout labour.

By the time I was pregnant with my third child, Jed, I was practising various birth positions and concentrating on squatting. I worked hard on my stiff ankles 10 minutes every day. Over many months the flexibility of my pelvis, knees and ankles gradually improved and I could adopt several birth positions with ease. During Jed's birth, I continued with my usual activities and even went for a swim in early labour. When the contractions grew strong, I followed my instincts and kept changing positions from squatting, to kneeling, to walking, resting when I felt like it and moving in any way that helped. To my surprise, the position I liked most was half-squatting and half-kneeling, on alternate legs. I took a bath and was kneeling on the floor in the all-fours position when the urge to push suddenly came. I stayed on all fours and pushed Jed out that way. He was a large, 9 lb baby. I had no tear, no grazes and a wonderful sense of control. I had, at last, given birth on my own two feet and was up and about with no soreness or stiffness at all after a day or two. Since then many of the women in my classes have asked me to recommend a book on preparing the body to adopt natural positions. Although most aspects of birth are well covered by the literature on the subject, there is no effective book as far as I know on preparing your body to adopt sensible, natural birth positions.

I hope that this book will fill the gap and that its contents will be as useful to you as they have been for me.

Janet Balaskas

My wife has taught women to prepare themselves for childbirth while I have taught men and women exercises that make their bodies supple and fit. Through our constant exchange of ideas, experiences and practices over the years, we decided to write this book of exercises for childbirth.

In writing **New Life** together, I feel we have made some additions to the existing teaching and literature on preparing for childbirth. Firstly, by emphasizing the relaxation of the body in action. To be able to relax deeply with the body at rest is not all there is to relaxation. The dynamic relaxation of a supple body is needed.

Secondly, by clearly showing *why* breathing is able to assist labour. To be taught when and how to breathe through the different contractions and stages of labour and not why is not good enough!

And thirdly, by encouraging a woman to know her own birth canal as much as she possibly can through her own touch. Unless a woman is in touch with the parts of her body through which her child will pass to be born how can she feel fully prepared for childbirth?

Furthermore, we are convinced of the importance of the following:

1   Recent research in South America, Spain and Britain (in Birmingham and Bristol) has suggested that it is physiologically better for a woman and her baby to keep upright and moving during the greater part of labour. The uterus contracts more effectively, the blood flow between placenta and child is better, pain is reduced and labour is shorter. They have shown clearly that when a woman stands, uterine contractions are 100% more efficient than when she lies down on her back or side.

2   The most commonly adopted postures of primitive women, which are also the most physiologically advantageous, involve being upright with a rounded out or curved back, hip joints flexed, knees bent and spread apart. It is in these inclining positions (as opposed to reclining positions) that the pelvis opens.

3   Radiographically it has been shown that the cross-sectional surface area of the birth canal may increase by as much as 30% when a woman changes from lying on her back to squatting.

In this book we have made two assumptions. The first is that, because the earliest, most primitive birth position is squatting, cultivating comfort and ease in squatting is the best preparation of the musculo-skeletal system of a woman's body for childbirth. And the second assumption is that, when the joints and muscles of the body function well, the body's maintenance and recuperative powers are enhanced — a well functioning musculo-skeletal system contributes greatly to physical well being and all-round health.

Arthur Balaskas

1 How to use this book

You are pregnant, but how are you to prepare for the feat of childbirth, both mentally and physically? You may not know how, and the purpose of this book is to show you what you need to do to be at your best when labour begins, both for your sake and for the sake of your child.

Pregnancy and childbirth are normal events and should be treated as such. At the same time, birth is one of the most strenuous activities of a woman's life, demanding great effort. Intelligent preparation can make it easier.

This book is not just a book to read, it is a book to participate in right from the start. The best plan is to read it straight through to begin with, in order to gain an overall picture of the processes of pregnancy and the preparations for childbirth.

However, on this first reading do follow the '*Try this*' advice with which the book is signposted. If you do, you will feel in your own body the sensations that are being described and you will understand them all the better.

After this preliminary reading, the purpose of the exercises will be clear and the time has come to begin practising them, first to become familiar with them and then gradually to grow at ease with them and enjoy them. The woman who perseveres is doing everything possible to be at her physical best when the day of labour arrives.

The sole aim of this book is to help the woman who is willing to work towards the birth of her child. It certainly does not set out to be a complete do-it-yourself guide to childbirth, for many people are likely to be involved in that, your doctor, obstetrician, midwife, ante-natal teacher and hospital staff. As soon as you are pregnant you should check the procedures, practices and choices offered. These vary from country to country, from town to town, from hospital to hospital, from obstetrician to obstetrician, and from midwife to midwife. You may be given the choice of giving birth at home or in hospital, or you may be given no choice. Your hospital may have the latest ultrasonic scanning facilities and biochemical monitoring, or it may not.

Every woman has to look into her local scene to get all the information she can. For instance, if you want to be active in labour and give birth in positions that suit you, you may find that your local G.P. or your local hospital are not entirely cooperative. If this is the case, you can contact the National Childbirth Trust, or the Birth Centre (London) and they will put you in touch with someone who may be able to help you.

In any case, you will probably take an ante-natal course and these usually begin towards the end of the seventh or the beginning of the eighth month of pregnancy. This training during the last phases of pregnancy keeps the methods and techniques involved fresh in the mind when actual labour begins. But physical preparation should begin long before, the sooner the better, preferably from the time you first know that you are pregnant or even when you feel that you would like to become pregnant. So, by the time you take an ante-natal course, your body should already be flexible and fit, with your pelvic organs, muscles, and joints in good condition. Even if your G.P. tells you that you are a 'special case', i.e., if you are having your first child, or you are past what is normally thought of as easy child-bearing age, or if you have had complications in previous deliveries, it is still definitely worth your while doing the exercises recommended in this book.

2 Your uterus

To understand what happens during pregnancy and childbirth you should know some simple facts about that part of your body in which your child is developing. The area is within your abdominal cavity (lower trunk). Your abdominal cavity extends from your diaphragm beneath your lungs to the muscles of the floor of your pelvis (1). Within the abdominal cavity lies your uterus, between the bladder in front and the rectum behind. It projects into the vagina almost at a right angle (2).

The uterus is the principal organ involved in pregnancy and childbirth. Your child is conceived in one of its fallopian tubes, implants within its wall, develops and grows within its cavity, and at the appropriate time is expelled by it through the vagina into the outside world (3).

In its non-pregnant state the uterus is a small, hollow muscular organ with the walls touching each other. It is divided into two parts, the uterine body and the cervix (neck) which projects into the vagina. At the beginning of pregnancy it measures roughly $3 \times 2 \times 1$ inches. During the forty weeks of pregnancy it increases greatly in size to contain the rapidly growing foetus until at the end it measures about $12 \times 9 \times 9$ inches. Its weight also increases from about 100 g to about 1000 g at full term.

During the first sixteen weeks of pregnancy the expansion of your uterus is caused almost entirely by the growth of its tissues owing to hormonal stimulation. The uterus becomes a thick-walled organ, circular in shape. From the twentieth week growth almost ceases and the uterus then expands because the muscle fibres are stretched by the growing child. The walls of the uterus become progressively thinner and in the latter half of pregnancy your child may easily be felt through these thin walls.

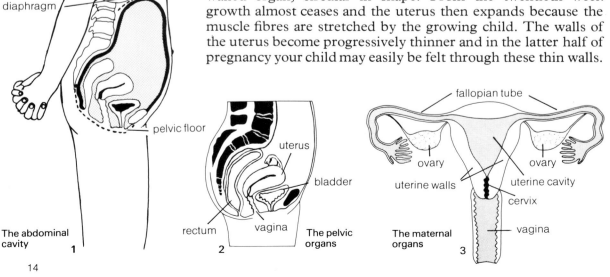

diaphragm

pelvic floor

uterus

bladder

rectum

vagina

fallopian tube

ovary

ovary

uterine walls

uterine cavity

cervix

vagina

The abdominal cavity 1

The pelvic organs 2

The maternal organs 3

The uterus becomes more oval in shape as your child grows up into your abdomen.

As your uterus enlarges, its position changes. It rises out of your pelvis and into contact with your abdominal wall. It remains in your pelvis until the end of the twelfth week when its upper part is just above the level of your pelvic inlet.

At the end of the sixteenth week its upper end is nearly half way to your navel, which it reaches at the end of the twenty-fourth week.

At thirty-six weeks its upper end is at the level of the lower end of your breastbone.

During the last few weeks it drops a little lower as your baby settles into position for birth.

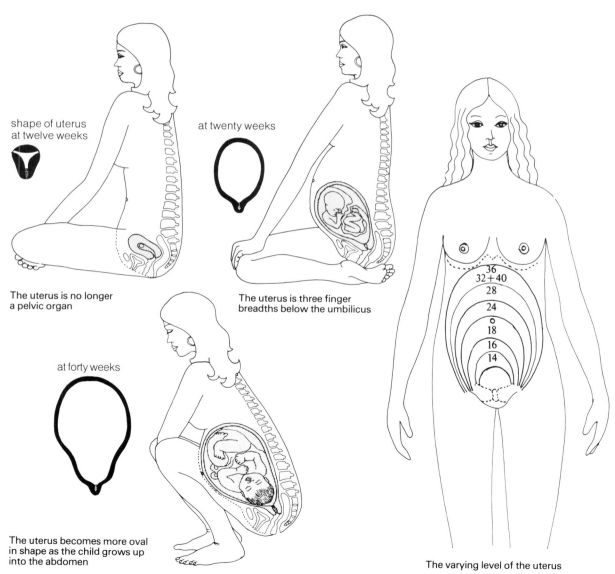

shape of uterus at twelve weeks

The uterus is no longer a pelvic organ

at twenty weeks

The uterus is three finger breadths below the umbilicus

at forty weeks

The uterus becomes more oval in shape as the child grows up into the abdomen

The varying level of the uterus

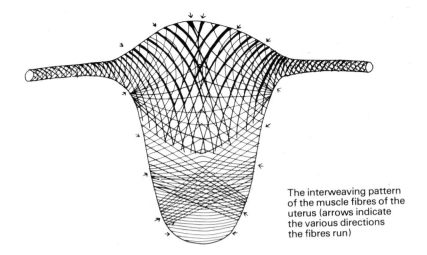

The interweaving pattern of the muscle fibres of the uterus (arrows indicate the various directions the fibres run)

The wall of the uterus consists of three coats or layers: (1) a surrounding covering coat (perimetrium); (2) a middle muscular coat (myometrium); (3) an inner mucous coat or lining (endometrium).

In childbirth it is the middle muscular layer that is the primary power behind the expulsion of your child.

The muscular part of the uterus is a network of muscle fibres and bundles running in all directions, longitudinal (lengthwise), oblique and circular, but in its expulsive action it functions as a single hollow muscular organ.

At full term, that is at the end of pregnancy, the function of your uterus is to evacuate its contents. This effort, known as labour, may be divided into three stages.

The first stage of labour

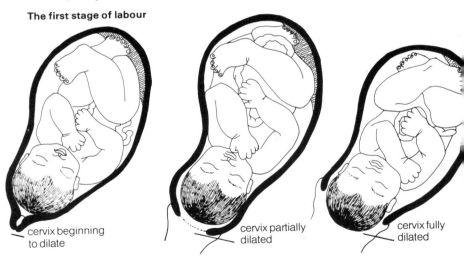

cervix beginning to dilate

cervix partially dilated

cervix fully dilated

The first stage is the stage of dilation, or opening of the cervix, which lasts from the onset of uterine contraction until the cervix is fully dilated. During pregnancy the cervix is progressively softened by the action of hormones and thus opens more readily during labour.

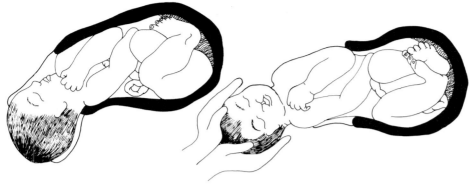

The second stage of labour

The second stage is the stage of expulsion and extends from complete dilation of your cervix to the expulsion – through the vagina – of your child. The walls of the vagina are capable of enormous stretching as your baby descends. Also, like your cervix, your vaginal walls have become softened during pregnancy.

This stage of labour is influenced by your will and voluntary effort, unlike the first stage, which is largely involuntary.

The third stage is the stage of the separation and expulsion of the placenta.

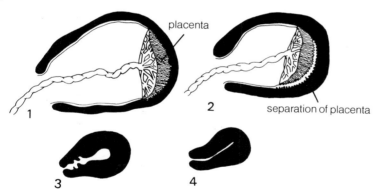

The third stage of labour

1 After the birth of the baby, the placenta remains in the uterus
2 The placenta loosens and separates from the uterine wall, and the uterus contracts to expel the placenta
3 The uterus shrinks gradually back into the pelvis by the second week after birth
4 The uterus returns to normal by the sixth week after birth

Expulsive organ

The uterus, like the neighbouring bladder and rectum within the abdominal cavity, is an expulsive organ. The muscular action of your uterus during labour in expelling your baby is similar to that of the other expulsive organs; some of the muscle fibres contract to reduce the size of each organ and others, which were keeping the outlet closed, relax to open it.

However, there is one vital difference. In childbirth (unlike menstruation, urination and defecation) your child has to go through not only the exit of the expulsive organ (your cervix and vagina) but also through the exit of your abdominal cavity, which is a narrow bony passage.

3 Your pelvic framework

To be born your child must pass through your pelvis, the girdle of bone that is the framework of the base and outlet of your trunk. Although, as we have seen in the last chapter, you have little conscious control over your uterus, you can control the working of your pelvic joints through your pelvic muscles. Because you can, by exercises and by practising various positions, increase the mobility of your pelvic framework during pregnancy and in labour, it is vital to understand the way in which it is built and how it works. You are greatly helped in this by being able to feel many of the pelvic bones and joints through your flesh, unlike the uterus which is a hidden and secret place.

Your pelvis is made up of four bones, the coccyx and sacrum wedged between two large hip bones. The hip bones are divided into three parts at birth, but fused at puberty. These are the iliac (flank or side), pubic (groin), and ischial (buttock) bones.

Take particular note of the pelvic joints. You will see that your sacrum joins your iliac bones at your sacroiliac joints, that your hips meet in front at your pubic joint and that your coccyx is attached to your sacrum at your sacrococcygeal joint. Besides these joints uniting your pelvis, the rest of your spinal column bears down on your sacrum at your lumbosacral joint with two smaller horn-like joints behind it, and your pelvis as a whole is supported by your thigh bones at your two hip joints.

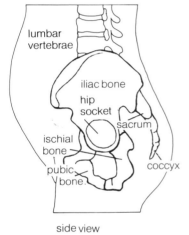

side view

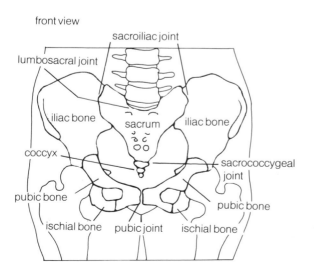

front view

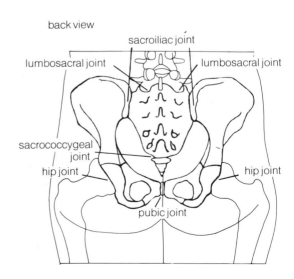

back view

To explore your pelvic bones *try this*. Feel the tangible parts of your iliac bones, which are the crests or tops of these bones. Feel the two bony knobs at the back end and the two in front. In the front of your pelvis feel the top pubic bones meeting in front. Using your thumbs and fingers, feel the top and bottom of your pubic joint; it is about one inch deep. Kneel down and locate the tips of your buttock bones. Running your fingers along these link them up to the bottom of your pubic joint. The arch you can feel is known as your subpubic arch. The diagram shows precisely where it is.

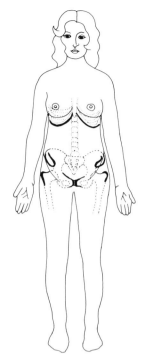

These two diagrams will help you to explore your pelvis. They show the tangible parts of the pelvis, the spine of the lower back, bottom ribs, and upper thighs

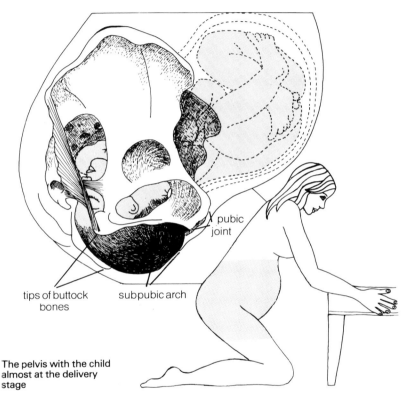

tips of buttock bones

subpubic arch

pubic joint

The pelvis with the child almost at the delivery stage

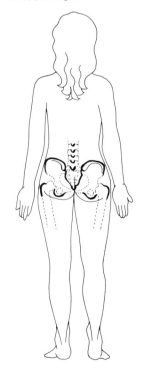

Place the palm of your hand over your sacrum with your fingers descending along to the tip of your coccyx. Touch and feel the back of your lower back (lumbar) vertebrae which rest on your sacrum. Stand up and feel the bony knobs on the outside of your thigh bones. These are often mistaken for your hip joints.

To explore your pelvic joints *try this*. Feel, touch, and explore your two tangible pelvic joints, the pubic and sacro-coccygeal joints. Now locate roughly the rest of your pelvic joints. The bony knobs at the back of your iliac crests cover and protect your sacroiliac and lumbosacral joints and the bony parts right at the front of your iliac crests are just above and protecting your two hip joints.

When moving your joints you either open or close them. The kind of movements possible at your hip joints are flexion (closing) and extension (opening), abduction (opening) and adduction (closing), and rotation inwards (closing) and rotation outwards (opening).

You will get the hang of all this by trying the simple movements in these self-explanatory diagrams.

The movements of the hip joint

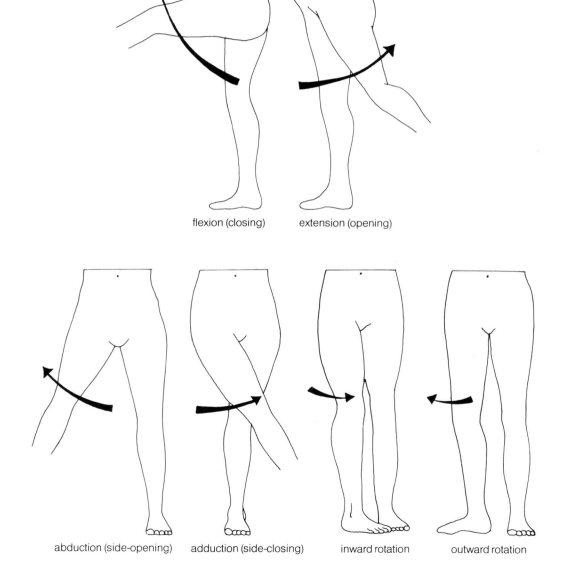

flexion (closing)   extension (opening)

abduction (side-opening)   adduction (side-closing)   inward rotation   outward rotation

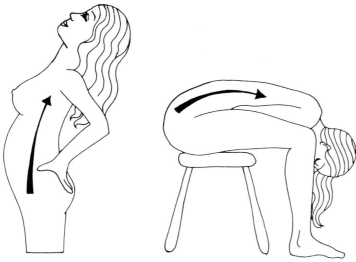

Extension of the trunk
(the front opens, the back closes)

Flexion of the trunk
(the back opens, the front closes)

When you extend your trunk the front part of your body opens and the back closes, whereas when you flex it the front closes and the back opens.

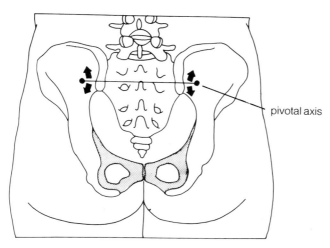

pivotal axis

The pivotal axis of the sacrum

Movements and changes of position possible at your pelvic joints

Your sacrum, which forms the back wall of your pelvis, is able to move slightly to and fro at its sacroiliac joints. From the diagram you can see that its pivotal axis is about one-third of its length from its top. This means that by flexing your trunk the outlet of your pelvic canal can be positioned to be opened, increasing its front-to-back distance.

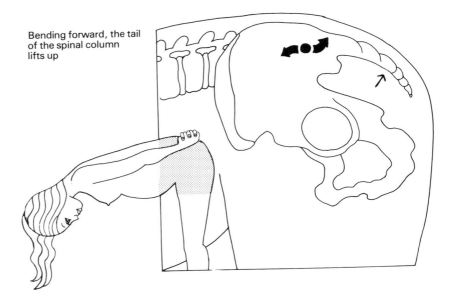

Bending forward, the tail of the spinal column lifts up

When the top part of your sacrum goes forward with your spinal column, the lower part extends backwards and opens (you lift your tail).

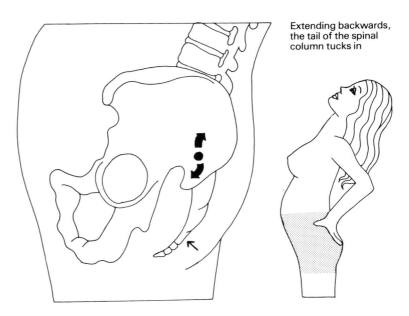

Extending backwards, the tail of the spinal column tucks in

When the top part of your sacrum goes backward with your spinal column, the lower part extends forwards and closes (you tuck in your tail).

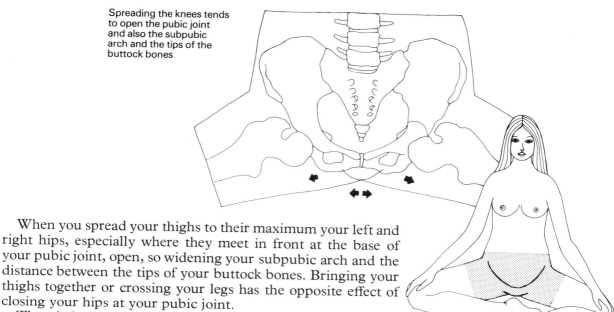

When you spread your thighs to their maximum your left and right hips, especially where they meet in front at the base of your pubic joint, open, so widening your subpubic arch and the distance between the tips of your buttock bones. Bringing your thighs together or crossing your legs has the opposite effect of closing your hips at your pubic joint.

The vital point is, that by flexing (bending forward) your trunk and abducting (spreading) your thighs, your pelvis is positioned at its widest and most opened, which is ideal for childbirth.

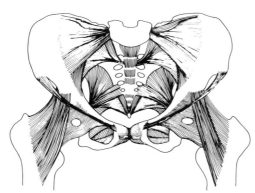

The ligaments of the pelvis

Ligaments

The bones of your pelvis are bound and held together at the joints by bands of tough, flexible, fibrous tissue called ligaments. They cannot be felt or touched, but the diagram will help you to visualize how they interweave and run in all directions. They are designed to prevent excessive or abnormal movements of the joints; each ligament becomes taut at its normal limit of some particular movement. During pregnancy a variety of hormones flow into the bloodstream causing these ligaments to swell, soften, and become more flexible in readiness for childbirth.

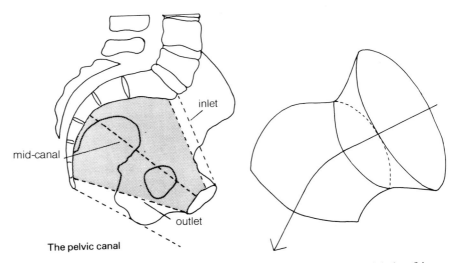

mid-canal

inlet

outlet

The pelvic canal

It will help you to understand your pelvis if you think of it as a curved funnel with an inlet, an outlet and a canal joining them. *Try this*: touch and feel the top of your pubic joint and part of the pubic bones on its sides; this is the only tangible part of the inlet. Now place one hand on your sacrum (the tips of your fingers on your coccyx) and place the thumb and fingers of your other hand on the top and bottom of your pubic joint. These two parts form the back and front walls of the pelvic canal, through which your child has to pass to be born.

Finally feel and explore the outlet of your pelvic canal, which is also the outlet of your lower trunk. To do this easily lie down with your feet on a chair. Feel your coccyx, the tips of your buttock bones, your subpubic arch and the base or bottom of your pubic joint. This is the outlet of your trunk through which your child finally passes to be born.

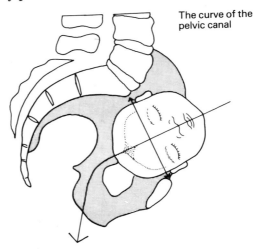

The curve of the pelvic canal

The pelvic canal is curved and your child's head must negotiate a sharp bend as it descends.

The pelvic canal inlet is wider from side to side than from front to back. The outlet is wider from front to back than from side to side. The differences are slight but, with the influence of the pelvic floor muscles, enough to force the child's head and body to rotate during descent. When your child's head enters the inlet the longest part is positioned from side to side and when it emerges through the outlet the longest part is positioned from front to back.

To become accustomed to this idea of your pelvis as a curved funnel through which your child must pass, it is very helpful and rewarding during pregnancy to touch and explore all the tangible parts of your bony birth canal, especially its outlet, when you take a bath or practise your exercises. Over the months this builds up an understanding of the process of birth and a sense of purpose during labour.

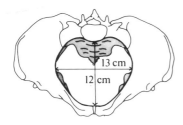

The inlet of the pelvis   The outlet of the pelvis

The female pelvis compared with the male
 (1) Female pelvic bones are lighter and smoother.
 (2) The iliac crests are further apart and the iliac bones more hollowed.
 (3) The sacrum is broader and its promontory less pronounced.
 (4) The pubic joint is less deep.
 (5) The pelvic inlet is larger, more oval, and less heart-shaped.
 (6) The canal is shallower and less funnel-shaped.
 (7) The pelvic canal's outlet is wider and the buttock bones further apart.
 (8) The pubic arch is wider (90° to 100°) than in the male (about 75°).
 (9) The coccyx is more movable.
(10) The hips sockets are further apart.

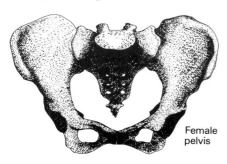
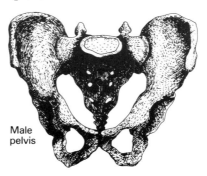

Female pelvis   Male pelvis

4 Your pelvic muscles

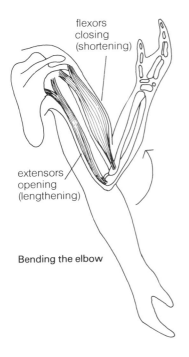

flexors
closing
(shortening)

extensors
opening
(lengthening)

Bending the elbow

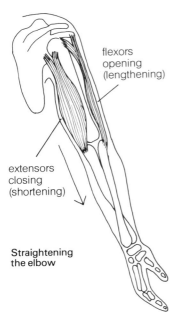

flexors
opening
(lengthening)

extensors
closing
(shortening)

**Straightening
the elbow**

About thirty-six pairs of muscles are attached to your pelvis and to appreciate their importance in childbirth it is essential to know a few basic facts about how muscles work.

How muscles work

If you think of bones as levers then muscles are the pulleys that support, position, and move the bones at their hinges, that is, the joints. Each joint is moved by two opposing teams of muscles, the flexors and the extensors. The action is simply demonstrated by bending your elbow.

When you straighten your arm, the extensors shorten and close behind and the flexors stretch and open in front. When you bend your elbow the flexors shorten and the extensors stretch.

It's like a tug of war, one team can gain only what the other loses. In short, muscles work joints in opposing yet complementary paired teams, when one team is fully shortening and closing, the other team is fully stretching and opening.

Another simple vital fact is that *all movements of bones at their joints are either resisted or assisted by gravity. Try this:* lie on your back and lift your head and trunk a little for a few seconds. The force of gravity resists the movement of your trunk and you sense your abdominal muscles tightening to shorten and pull your trunk upwards. Now stand up with your legs apart and bend forward towards your toes with back and knees straight. Gravity assists the movement of your trunk with no tightening of your abdominal muscles. Now you sense your back thigh muscles – especially behind your knees – stretching and opening, perhaps even painfully.

Pelvic muscles

Keeping in mind how muscles work in pairs and the importance of gravity in our movements we can look closely at the pelvic muscles. From the pelvis they run up to your neck and head, down through your thighs, all about and through your abdominal wall, and enclosing the outlet of your pelvis. In this way most of the large and powerful muscles of your body are drawn together under the control of your pelvis. They make up most of the muscles of your lower trunk and your upper thighs. *Try this:* with the help of the diagram, roughly locate with your hands all the tangible muscle groups attached to your pelvis, your abdominal, lower back, buttock, upper thigh muscles, and those enclosing the outlet of your pelvis. There are also other deeper muscles that cannot be felt.

The muscles that govern the two movements illustrated in the preceding chapter, that is, flexion of your trunk and abduction of your thighs, involve almost all your pelvic muscles in some way. These two movements position your pelvis at its widest extent.

Movement 1: Flexion of your trunk and thighs

The team of muscles that shorten in flexion of your trunk and thighs are called the flexors and the opposing team that stretch are the extensors.

Try this: sitting on the edge of your chair lower your chest towards your thighs. The shortening and closing team of muscles (flexors) are those in front of your body. These are being assisted by gravity and the stretching and opening team (extensors), also assisted by gravity, are those at the back of your body.

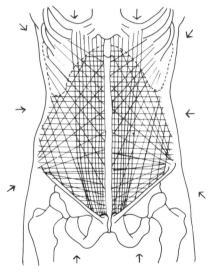

The interweaving pattern of the muscle fibres of the abdomen. (The arrows indicate the different directions in which they run)

Flexor muscles of the trunk and thighs are tangible

abdominal muscles

upper thigh muscles

The flexors of your trunk and thighs

These include three groups of muscles in front of your body.

Your abdominal muscles, which are made up of four layers, longitudinal, external slanting, side-to-side and internal slanting groups. Stroke your abdomen in the direction of these four layers trying to visualize them. These muscles are of great importance in childbirth because they are the main muscles bearing down on your uterus to aid its expulsion in the second stage of labour.

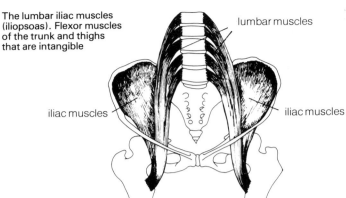

The lumbar iliac muscles (iliopsoas). Flexor muscles of the trunk and thighs that are intangible

lumbar muscles

iliac muscles

iliac muscles

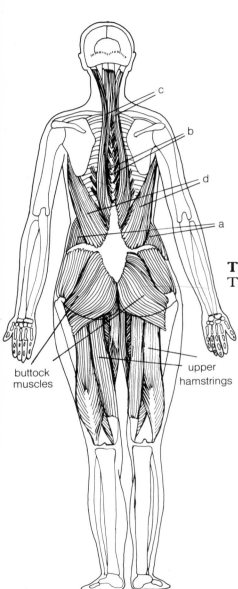

c

b

d

a

buttock muscles

upper hamstrings

The back muscles attached to the pelvis. These all lengthen when the trunk and thighs are flexed

Your lumbar-iliac muscles work in harmony with your abdominal muscles. When they shorten and contract, as in squatting, they bend your spinal column, pelvis, and thighs forwards. From the diagram visualize them roughly in your own body; they lie deep within and cannot be felt.

Your front upper thigh muscles, the third group in the team of trunk and thigh flexors, also serve to flex your pelvis towards your thighs when they contract.

The extensors of your trunk and thighs

These include four groups of muscles at the back of your body.

Your lower back muscles, shown in the diagram, are: (a) the muscles connecting your lower ribs to the crests of your iliac bones; (b) muscles that extend from your spinal column to your chest, neck and head; (c) muscles connecting your sacrum to the back of your head; (d) superficial muscles forming the broadest muscles of your back from your sacrum, lower back, and spinal column to your arms.

Try this: stand up and place your thumbs into the sides of your iliac bones with your fingers on the sides of your spinal column. Now walk and you will feel them alternately contract and stretch. When you bend forward, as in crouching, these muscles stretch and open and are assisted by gravity. When you bend back they contract and close.

Your buttock muscles. With the help of the diagram, feel your buttock muscles. These are the largest voluntary muscles in your body and are mainly responsible for the movement of your sacrum and coccyx (base of your spinal column) and the back wall of your pelvic canal and, most importantly, the back wall of its outlet. These, too, will stretch and open when you bend forward and will tighten when you lean back.

Your upper back thighs (hamstrings). From the diagram locate these muscles with your hands.

Try this: stand up with legs slightly apart and knees straight. Lean forward, keeping your back straight, while touching these upper hamstring muscles. You can feel them stretching as they are assisted by gravity.

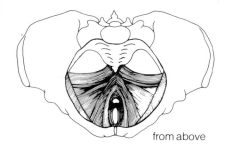
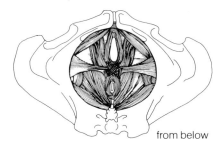
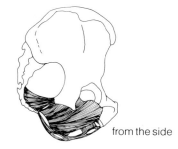

from above   from below   from the side

The pelvic floor

Your pelvic floor muscles. Sit comfortably, legs apart with your back supported. Locate the muscles that enclose your pelvic outlet, they extend from your lower sacrum and coccyx at the back, across your buttock bones and subpubic arch to your pubic joints in front. These muscles form the floor of your pelvis and lower trunk, supporting their contents. Two layers of muscles make up this floor; the deeper inner layer is known as the pelvic diaphragm and the outer the perineal muscles. What happens to the pelvic floor in childbirth is explained in detail in the sections on squatting and labour.

Movement 2: Abduction of thighs and hips
The two teams of muscles involved in this movement are the inner adductors and the outer abductors of the thighs. Your adductors run from your pubic bones to the insides of your thighs. These muscles may be roughly located with your hands. Lie against the wall with legs apart (see page 45). Feel your inner thigh adductors, they are stretching and opening in this position and allow your legs to open. When your legs are closed the outer thigh muscles (abductors) allow you to close your legs. These muscles on the sides of your hips run from your outside iliac bones down the outsides of your thighs to your knees.

When you open your thighs (e.g. in the squatting position) your abductors are shortening and your adductors are stretching, opening the outlet of your trunk from side to side. Your left hip goes to the left and your right hip goes to the right.

Summary
Remember that the action of your uterus in labour is purely involuntary. In labour, especially in the second expulsive stage, your uterus is assisted by the voluntary muscles of the lower trunk. By understanding the actions of these voluntary muscles and adopting sensible postures for birth, you can help to ensure that there will be adequate expansion of your pelvis so that your baby can take the line of least resistance. The point of physical preparation for childbirth is to get the muscles of your lower trunk in the best possible condition during the months before labour begins.

5 Relaxation

Although the importance of relaxation in labour and childbirth is widely recognized, the nature of bodily relaxation is not often properly understood, and the means of cultivating it are often limited and ineffectual.

What is relaxation?

You cannot know the nature of muscle relaxation without knowing the nature of muscle contraction, and the best and simplest way to investigate both is to examine them in your own body.

Just sitting and reading these words depends on a series of muscle contractions and relaxations. When you swallow, fidget, move your legs and arms, or just sit upright – no matter what – muscles are contracting and relaxing to make these movements possible. Most of these muscle contractions and relaxations do not reach consciousness, but there are times when muscles contract or relax sufficiently for you to be aware of them.

Muscle contraction

The moment any part of your body meets resistance, muscle contraction takes place.

Try this: lift up the edge of a table an inch or two with your fingers. You can feel the muscles of your arm tighten and contract. The weight of the table is offering resistance to the movement of your arm. In fact, resist any movement enough and immediately you will be aware of muscles tightening or hardening or going rigid, giving rise to a feeling of tension.

Muscle relaxation

Muscles relax when the range of movement or position of your body or any part of it is extreme enough and is felt as stretching.

Try this: stand up and extend your arms overhead and simulate a yawn. Or stand with your legs slightly apart and knees straight, and bend (keeping your back straight) towards the floor. In both these instances you will feel muscles stretching, that is, relaxing and lengthening. When your hands go over your head you experience a stretch in front of your chest and arms and when you touch the floor you may feel the backs of your legs, especially behind your knees, stretching. If these muscles are stiff it may be painful.

When you make any movement or when you sit and read or

talk or walk, muscle groups are alternately contracting and relaxing. Indeed, all bodily tissues are subject to this rhythm. It is the principle of work pairing rest. As one part or system contracts it throws its working partner into a phase of relaxation.

Contraction and relaxation of your muscles are so timed and graded in force that their combined actions and reactions maintain your body's postures and movements in space at all times.

Muscle contraction uses energy, relaxation does not

When muscles contract they use up energy and liberate heat. The amount of heat freed is the measure of energy used. When you run or exert yourself in any activity that demands much muscle contraction, your body soon gets hot. Another example of the way muscle contraction uses energy and frees heat is the phenomenon of shivering when cold. Muscles involuntarily contract, making small movements and creating heat to increase your body temperature.

On the other hand, when muscles relax they do not use energy or liberate heat. They can relax in two ways.

By resting. When they have no resistance to overcome, i.e. no work to do, they are then inactive both in terms of energy and mechanically. **By stretching**. They are resting at their maximum length and are then inactive in terms of energy, but mechanically active.

You will appreciate this distinction by these examples.

1 If you lie down comfortably with your legs together and at rest, your inner thigh muscles will be relaxed and resting (mechanically inactive without using energy). 2 If you lie with your legs apart on the wall, you are, mechanically speaking, lengthening your inner thigh muscles to allow your legs to widen to their maximum. These muscles are mechanically stretched to their maximum but are in a state of passive relaxation (i.e. they are not using up energy).

The use of willpower in relaxation

Try this: stop reading for a few moments. Get up from your sitting position, lie on the floor for a few seconds and return to sitting and reading. Do this before reading on. If you ask yourself how you did this, you will realize that you merely willed yourself to stop reading, to lie down, and to return to reading. You just did it. You made the decision to do it and went ahead. You did not concern yourself whether muscles were contracting or relaxing, which part to move first and so on. You just willed and it all happened.

Postures and movements of your body are voluntary, whether you are aware of it or not. To move or position your body or any part of it involves the decision or will to do so. When you bend forward, you merely will it and it happens. You don't concern yourself with your hips or the muscles of your legs and back and so on. So, although movement and posture are directly controlled by the will, muscles are only indirectly controlled; they can never be willed to contract or relax. Even the control of your face is indirect and it is just the same with your pelvic floor. You can control only the opening and closing of different orifices, and not the muscles themselves.

Through your will you can assume a position in which your body is well supported and at rest. This renders your muscles inactive and inoperative and provides relaxation by resting the muscles. Also through your will you can assume an extreme position or make an extreme movement in which some of your joints are at the limit of their range (e.g. fully flexing or fully extending). This gives relaxation by stretching muscles.

A movement step by step

Normally the mistaken idea that muscles can contract and relax at will (as if muscles can be switched on and off) does not matter. But in labour and childbirth, when relaxation by resting and stretching skeletal muscles is crucial, such a misapprehension is misleading. You need to know the location of the parts of your pelvis to be moved and in what direction these parts may be moved to expand the outlet of your pelvis.

To relax by stretching your pelvic-floor muscles in the second stage of labour involves willing your pelvis to open in a particular manner – that is, from front to back and from side to side, as it does when making the movements of squatting or kneeling. This has to be willed in order that muscles stretch and relax. Again, in order that your abdominal muscles contract efficiently, you have to will your abdominal cavity to close.

Women are often advised to relax certain muscles, such as those of the pelvic floor or thighs. But this can be done only through moving your body or opening and closing its orifices by the use of your will. You can't directly relax your pelvic-floor muscles by ordering them to relax. It's confusing to try. It's like asking someone to relax their eyelid muscles so that their eyes will open.

How is relaxation cultivated?

As we have seen, muscles relax when they are resting or stretching. Resting muscles allows them to recuperate. Stretching muscles revitalizes them.

Unwittingly or not, you are constantly relaxing your muscles by resting and stretching them. These are inborn skills, and the cultivation of relaxation involves developing them to your best advantage. Animals relax their muscles in the same ways. Watch a cat sleeping, resting, and stretching and you will marvel at the ease with which it does so. The rudimentary techniques for cultivating relaxation are simply the ordered and organized resting and stretching of muscles in appropriate bodily positions or postures.

Cultivation of resting

In a supported position you may be able to rest all your muscles completely, or you may find it difficult, or you may think you can but in fact can't completely. If you cannot take it for granted, you may need to cultivate resting in preparation for childbirth and as a supplement to sleep. A few minutes a few times a day, especially after exertion, will work wonders. It is not always easy to do at first, but like so many other skills it becomes easier with practice.

Resting positions

Any position of your body whereby its parts are supported, thus rendering your skeletal muscles inoperative and inactive, is appropriate for resting. The three most useful positions are:
1 lying down on your back – this is the simplest position and can be helpful during pregnancy, but should be avoided in the last month or if you feel uncomfortable lying on your back. (See **Caution** on page 37.); **2** sitting on a chair resting your arms and head on a table or sitting facing backwards on a chair leaning on the back for support; **3** sitting on your feet, kneeling, with knees slightly apart and your arms and head resting on a chair or low table or bed.

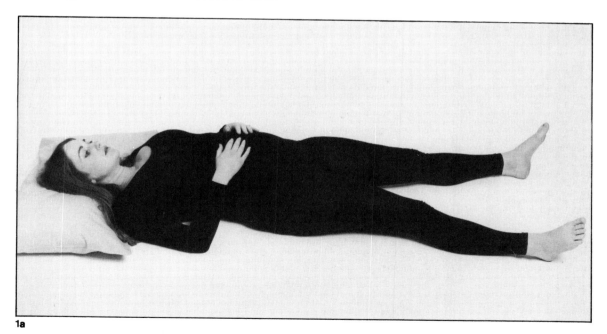

1a

Resting exercises

Position 1: Lie down on a firm surface (**1a**). If your entire spinal column, including your lower back, rests on the floor the position is an effortless one for you. If your lower back does not touch the floor use a cushion and a chair (**1b** next page).

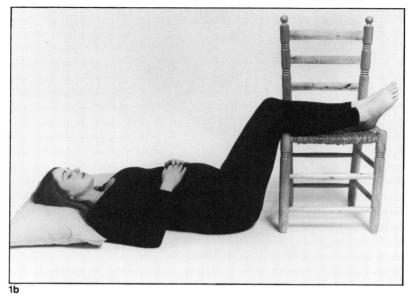

1b

In order to render your muscles inactive each part of your
body should be independently supported. When you lie on your
back on the floor, your feet, ankles, hips, thighs, pelvis, trunk,
shoulders, arms, wrists, hands, neck, and head should be
independently supported by the floor. Proper support for each
part of your body is the first essential for resting muscles in
order to make them inoperative and inactive.

Position 2: If you are upright, amd more so when you are
inclining or crouching, gravity aids the body of your uterus to
push down on your baby and so open the neck of your uterus.
A way of resting in an upright leaning-forward position during
the first stage of labour is needed. Lean over the table or on the
back of your chair and rest your head on your arms or on a
cushion (2). Let your shoulders, arms, and trunk slacken, resting
fully on the table, and let your thighs fall apart. Each part of
your body should be supported directly or indirectly by the
chair and table, or whatever you are sitting and leaning on. If
your bed is high enough, you can use a stool or a low chair to sit
on and lean on the bed. Remember that proper support is
always the first essential for resting muscles and for giving them
no work to do.

This resting position is very helpful during the first stage of
labour, so it is beneficial to get used to it. It is similar to
squatting; in both positions your ankles, knees, hips, back, and
neck are all flexed, your thighs spread apart (abducted), and you
are on your own two feet. Resting in such a position, well-
supported and comfortable, minimizes muscle activity. Support
of your body in such a way can be as complete as when your
body is fully reclined, as long as your legs are apart to allow
resting of all your inner thigh muscles.

Position 3: In the first stage and in the expulsive second stage of labour when bearing-down positions are used, a convenient and comfortable position to rest your body between uterine contractions is needed.

Step 1: sit on your feet or on a cushion between your feet, and with knees easily apart lean and rest your head on your arms or on a cushion placed on a low table or chair or bed (**3**).

After assuming resting position

You may still have to learn to let go when in these three resting positions. This may seem surprising since it might be supposed that in such positions you cannot be anything but relaxed.

Step 2: whichever position you are in, take a few deep breaths or sigh deeply from way down in your abdomen. With eyes open or closed, become aware of how you feel, not whether you are happy or depressed or bored, but the actual sense of feeling in various parts of your body.

As though it were an exploration into the unknown, feel from within all parts of your body. Start with your face, hands, and then your feet and finally your eyes. It should be done without effort, a gentle moving awareness of the different parts of your body and then of your body as a whole. The whole secret of

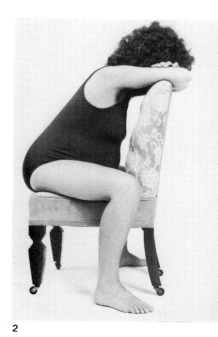

2

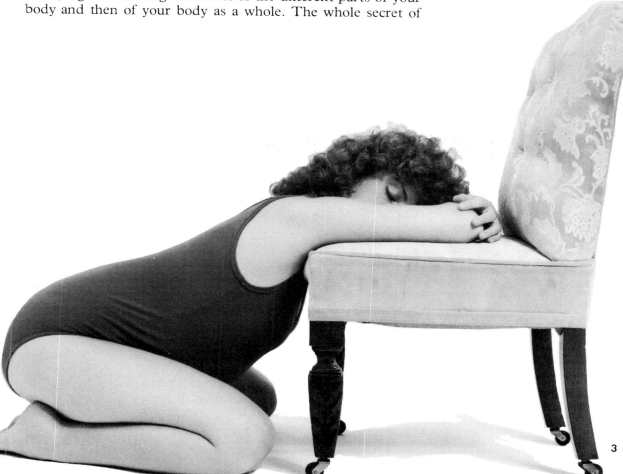

3

successful resting is to be in an appropriate resting position and fully aware of your body.

Focusing attention on your body and its parts is a means of stopping you thinking and worrying. It is also the means of localizing tightness or slight muscle contractions.

You can learn with practice to recognize the slight but definite sensations that are always present when muscles are tightened or tensed (contracted). Then, when you have learnt to appreciate this slight tightening, you can train yourself to stop it by willing your body to surrender its resistance to the resting position. (Remember that you can't relax muscles by willpower like switching off a light, but you can use your will to let go of unnecessary tension or resistance.)

As a further aid to stopping thinking, special attention may be paid to the resting of muscles used in thinking. Muscles of your eyes and of speech are used as much for thinking as they are for seeing and speaking. Your tongue, jaw, eyes, forehead, nose, and lips have a larger area of your brain allocated to their sensory and motor activity than does any other part of your body.

For this reason, it is reasonably easy to feel the sensations of these parts and so cease any movements or expression of your face, thus resting the muscles involved. When your face is moving or holding an expression your facial muscles contract strongly. Other areas of your body may quickly be affected and muscles in these other parts tend to contract in sympathy. It is very difficult to rest the remainder of your body when your facial muscles are strongly contracted.

If you can keep your face relaxed in the first stage of labour, it helps tremendously to maintain a state of relaxation in the rest of your body.

Your hands are your next most sensitive part, they come second in the brain area allocated to them. It is usually easy to rest them and this should be done after resting your face.

Repeat Step 2: focus your attention on your face and let it become expressionless. Then on your hands, make sure they are loose. Then your toes; let them go loose. Then on your ankles; let your feet go slack. Do the same with your knees, thighs, buttocks, and the base of your pelvis. Continue in this way, focusing awareness on each area in turn until every part of your legs, trunk, shoulders, arms, hands, neck, and face are resting.

Five to ten minutes of complete resting in such positions (reclining or supported sitting) is extremely valuable during pregnancy, especially if you are tired or tense and unable to take a long rest. If you are too tired or tense to sleep, the practice of resting lying on your back may lead to sound sleep.

Resting when you are comfortable without any stress is quite different from doing it during uterine contractions. However, it is possible, during the first stage of labour, in a well-supported position, to rest your skeletal system (bones, joints, and muscles) while all that activity is happening within you. The only way to cultivate the ability to carry resting into full effect during labour is through practice and in this way you may help yourself through pregnancy as well.

Caution: during pregnancy, particularly in the last few weeks, some women experience dizziness when lying on their backs. This is due to a slowing in the circulation caused by pressure from the weight of the uterus on the external blood vessels. If you are affected in this way lie on your side instead, with cushions supporting your head and knee.

Cultivation of stretching

If any joints in your body are stiff, you need to improve the ability to stretch and relax the muscles governing them.

There are stiff joints and relatively unrelaxable muscles governing them throughout your body, even though you may not be directly aware of them. Stiffness is chronic (i.e. continually present) and mostly hidden. By unwittingly reducing the range of your activities (i.e. your range of movements at joints) you may avoid noticing your stiffness.

If you normally sit, stand, walk, run a little, drive, lie down, rest, and sleep and not much more, then your stiffness may not be apparent to you. Only when you extend yourself, when you extend the range of movements at your joints, are you in a position to judge whether these joints and the muscles governing them are stiff or not. There is no other way for shortened, stiff muscles to regain their elasticity and relaxability other than through their gradual stretching over a period of time.

The more stiff or rigid your muscles, the more difficult will be your task in gradually stretching them. But remember that during pregnancy nature automatically increases your suppleness and stretching muscles is therefore easier.

Stretching a group of muscles goes one step further than resting them. Resting them is freeing them from work or activity and so no energy is used, but stretching demands this and more; it demands the complete release of resistance in order to gain the length or expansion necessary to allow the full movement or position. Squatting and positions complementary to it are basically organized stretching of muscles, as opposed to instinctive stretching which happens automatically.

The most important specific groups of muscles needed to be relaxed and stretched in childbirth are the muscles of your pelvic floor, buttocks, and thighs. During the expulsive stage of labour these are the central skeletal muscles involved, whereas the rest of your skeletal muscles are peripheral.

Cultivation of resting and stretching the major muscles of your body is perhaps the greatest aid to relaxation during labour.

6 Exercises

During pregnancy it is perfectly safe to lead an active normal life and to move about much as usual. Of course you may have to cut out excessively strenuous activities such as skating or horse jumping. Also, as pregnancy progresses, you will tend to slow down considerably, partly because of the extra weight you carry and partly because of caution. Many women have been erroneously told that if you stretch or bend or simply move too much you will somehow injure your baby. This is untrue. If you enjoy swimming, tennis, golf, walking or gardening you should continue to do these until they become uncomfortable and too much for you.

In addition to these normal activities there are special exercises that should be done to prepare you for childbirth. Obviously these are different exercises from those you would do to improve your performance in running a mile, swimming a hundred metres, riding a horse, or playing tennis. In childbirth you don't need to run a mile or swim twenty lengths and so on. You need to have flexible joints and relaxable muscles.

Labour is a great muscular feat that requires the dynamic use of your joints, ligaments, tendons, and muscles. The nucleus of this activity involves roughly the area immediately above your pelvis and immediately below it. This is the part of your body that should be exercised and improved in flexibility and relaxability.

More specifically what you have to practise is the expansion of the pelvic joints, the relaxation of the pelvic floor, the closing of the abdominal cavity, and the contraction of the abdominal wall.

Many women have stiff pelvic joints. Much can be done to overcome this by exercising these joints in squatting and other positions. Happily, the joints automatically become slightly more flexible during pregnancy and this is a help in getting rid of stiffness.

Although it is never too late, the best time to begin practising exercises is not a month or two before labour, but from the time when you first know you are pregnant.

The type of exercise suitable for pregnancy must first of all not be strenuous or tiring. It should save energy and release unnecessary muscle tension. Second, the exercises should improve the sensitivity of your body's joints and muscles and your awareness of them.

The effect of exercises on breathing and circulation is particularly important. With vigorous or prolonged exercise the speed of circulation and depth of breathing are increased, your heart beating more quickly and forcefully. *Exercises to be done during pregnancy should, therefore, be carefully chosen.* They should be non-strenuous, passive, and reduce your heart beat and breathing rate. They should bring energy rather than use it up, and always be assisted by gravity rather than resisted by it. This can be achieved by the position in which the body is placed for an exercise, for example, squatting. (Any exercise that is determined merely by the position of the body may be described as a positional exercise.)

What to avoid

Avoid rigid physical jerks, strenuous, complicated or very athletic exercises. Avoid exercises that demand you move against gravity, such as straight leg lifting on your back, and those that involve deep hollowing of the small of your back.

Do not lie on your back and lift both legs or raise your trunk up to a sitting position without the aid of your arms. Do not perform exercises that are strenuous enough to make you hold your breath. This strains your abdominal muscles.

Initial discomfort

When you try these positions for the first time, you may not be able to do them fully or you may find them rather painful. You may fear that the initial discomfort indicates that they are risky, injurious or harmful. But every new physical activity or exercise begins with some discomfort, as when you take up a game you haven't played for years. The exercises and positions demand muscle relaxation and stretching, and it may be painful at first to be forced to relax and alter muscular habits because breaking any habit is difficult.

Don't let the initial discomfort put you off. You are suffering because your joints and muscles have temporarily lost their full flexibility and elasticity. Through the various positions you are gently and gradually encouraging your joints and muscles to give up their habitual stiffness. The discomfort or pain are signs that joints and muscles are regaining their lost sensitivity. In time the initial disagreeable sensations gradually change into pleasure. Even from the very beginning, you will feel more relaxed after doing these exercises.

The following list of exercises includes: **1** instructions for carrying them out; **2** reasons for doing them, since it doesn't make sense to do them without knowing why; **3** recommendations about the time to be spent on them; and suggestions about when they may conveniently be done. Some may be done while having a bath, shower or wash. Some may be done at any time, or just before going to sleep; others need a set time each day when you won't be disturbed. A few exercises need the help of a partner and many are more satisfying if a friend or husband will practise them with you. The ideal set-up for many women is practising with two or three people, maybe friends who are also pregnant or who wish someday to become pregnant and see the good sense in overcoming stiff pelvic joints and muscles.

Caution: during pregnancy, particularly in the last weeks, some women experience dizziness when lying on their backs. This is due to a slowing in the circulation caused by pressure from the weight of the uterus on the internal blood vessels. If you are affected in this way omit all the postures which involve reclining and concentrate on the others.

Exercise 1: Sitting on your heels with knees apart
Sit on your heels and spread your knees comfortably apart. If this is difficult use a cushion to start with (**1a, b**). As a variation lean forward on your hands or elbows (**1c**).

How you benefit : the most common sites of stiffness are your knees and ankles. Gravity assists your ankles to extend and open and your knees to flex and close. The main muscles stretched and relaxed are those in the front of your lower legs and ankles. The variation flexes and closes your hip joints and extends and opens your pelvic outlet from front to back.

Time : at the start stay sitting on your heels for one minute and build up to five to ten minutes. Set time daily, undisturbed. Alternatively, this position and many others can be done while watching T.V., listening to music or reading, and need no extra time.

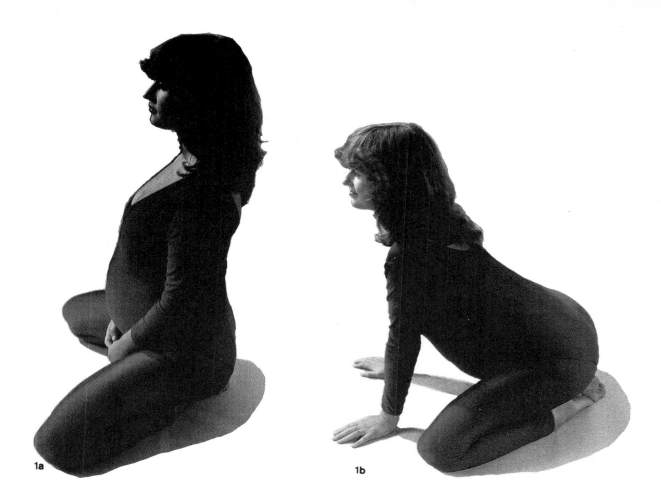

1a

1b

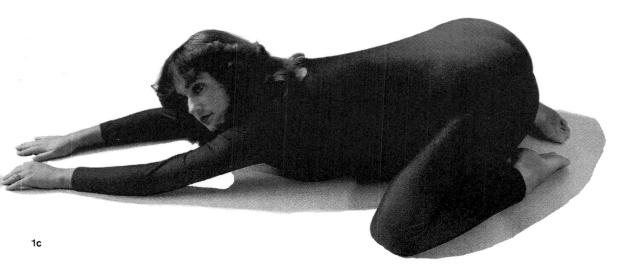

1c

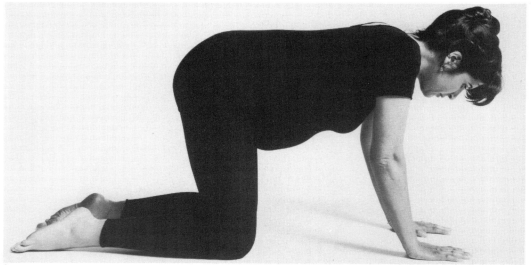

2a

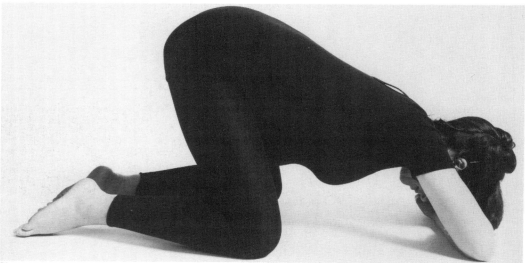

2b

Exercise 2: All-fours position

Sit on your heels. Bend forwards on to your hands and spread your knees comfortably apart. Keep your back as easy and straight as possible, that is, make sure your chest is not too close or too far from your pelvis (**2a**). As a variation, bend your elbows and place your forearms with the palms of your hands on the floor. Now rest your head gently on the floor (knee–chest position **2b**).

How you benefit: the position takes the load of weight off your sacrum and often relieves acute backache. It is also a balanced, ground-level position during labour – especially during the final stages.

Time: stay in the position and the variation for two to three minutes each. Set time daily, undisturbed.

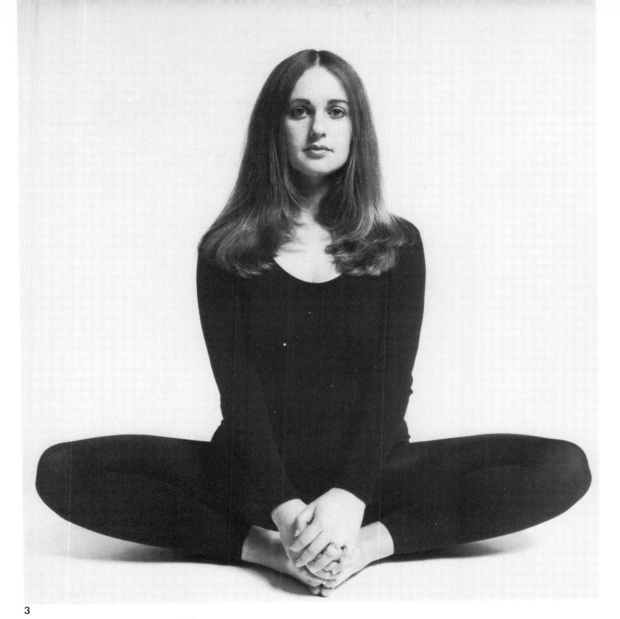

3

Exercise 3: Tailor position
Sit on the floor with your legs stretched out in front of you.
Bend your knees and at the same time bring the soles of your
feet together. Grip your feet and bring them as close to your
groin as possible. Widen your thighs and lower your knees as
far as you can on to the floor (**3**). Try to sit upright by sitting on
the front of your buttock bones and not on the back of them. If
this is difficult, sit on a cushion or lean against a wall to straighten
and ease your back. To help your knees down you may gently
push your thighs down with your elbows. You can also lift your
thighs slightly and drop them in rhythm, building up
momentum.

The most common fault in this sitting position is that your
trunk falls back because you are not sitting on the front of your

buttock bones. At first you may experience aches or pains in your knees, inner thighs or groin. This position demands the stretching of your inner thighs and if they are unable to relax sufficiently your knees cannot touch the floor. In time and with practice their stiffness can be reduced.

How you benefit: in this position your knees are flexed and closed, your hip joints are abducted, outwardly rotated and opened and your pubic joint is opened, your pubic arch and buttock bones are also separated and opened. Gravity again assists these joint positions so that the muscles governing your knee and hip joints, especially your inner thigh muscles and groin, are resting and stretching and are therefore relaxed.

Cultivation of this position increases the flexibility of your knee and hip joints, and the muscles governing them lose their stiffness and are made more relaxable.

Time spent: start with one minute and increase to five to ten minutes. Set time daily, undisturbed. Get into the habit, if possible, of sitting in this position when watching T.V. or talking to friends.

Exercise 4: Tailor position on a wall
Lie on your back with your buttocks against a wall and your legs straight. Bend your knees and bring your feet to meet each other, taking your knees as close to the wall as possible (**4**).

How you benefit: this is a resting position as the force of gravity assists the positions of your joints.

Time: stay in this position for one or two minutes and build up your time to five minutes. Set time daily, undisturbed.

4

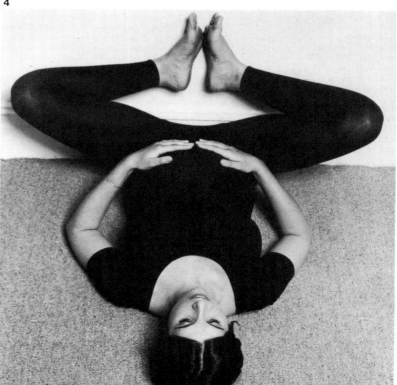

Exercise 5: Legs apart on a wall

Lie on your back with your buttocks against a wall and your legs straight on the wall. Slowly spread your legs apart as far as they will comfortably go. Keep your knees extended, but not tight, and do not point your toes (5). This simple position, aided by the force of gravity, lengthens, stretches, and opens your inner thigh muscles. The stiffer the muscles, the less wide your legs will spread. Initially aches and pains are experienced, mostly where these muscles meet your knees.

How you benefit : because your hip joints are abducted and opened to their maximum, your pubic joint, and thus your pubic arch and buttock bones, are separated and opened from side to side. This is a very good position for exploring the bones and muscles of your pelvic outlet, especially your pubic arch.

This position also helps in the relief of varicose veins. Sometimes the blood circulation becomes slower in the later months of pregnancy, especially after long standing, as when shopping. The veins have too much blood in them and they swell, their walls become thin and the valves do not quite close. The sluggishness of the circulation caused by pressure on the large veins in the pelvis and abdomen may also cause haemorrhoids or piles. All the postural exercises for the ankles, knees, and hips assist and encourage circulation of the blood and help to avoid these conditions.

Tired and swollen legs may be relieved by resting with your pelvis and legs elevated above your heart. Elevation of your legs allows the venous blood to flow into your body by the action of gravity. The relaxation, expansion, and stretching of the

5

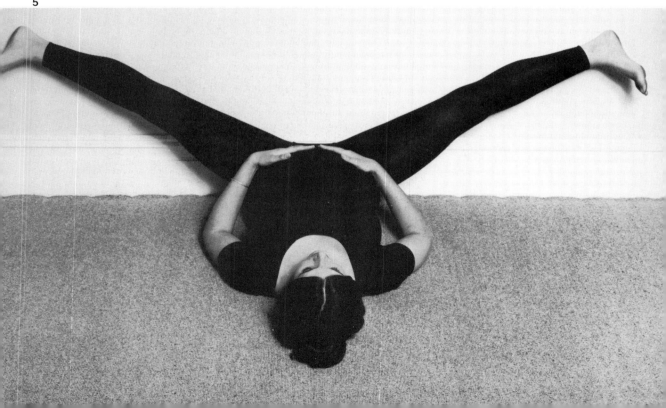

adductor muscles, in which the largest of these veins are located, means that blood is flowing into them. Massage of your thighs in this legs apart position, in the form of kneading, stretching, and squeezing, is of great benefit.

Time : start with half a minute in the legs-apart-on-a-wall position and gradually build up to five minutes. Set time daily, undisturbed.

Exercise 6: Squatting on a wall

Lie on your back with your buttocks against a wall and your legs on the wall. Spread your feet slightly and bend your knees and hips as if you were squatting on the wall. Your toes should be turned slightly outwards and heels flat on the wall. Now take your arms overhead, hands extended and your elbows straight and firm (**6**). Avoid struggling or lifting up your shoulders as your arms lie overhead. For most people this position is reasonably easy and comfortable, but to begin with you may experience aches and pains in your shoulders or groin. As your arms are extended overhead, your pectoral or breast muscles are stretched and relaxed (overcoming their stiffness). There is no muscle tissue in your breasts, but their tissues are continued to your breastbone, collar bones and shoulders and they are attached very firmly over most of the surfaces of your pectoral muscles. These strong elastic, fan-shaped muscles suspend your breasts

6

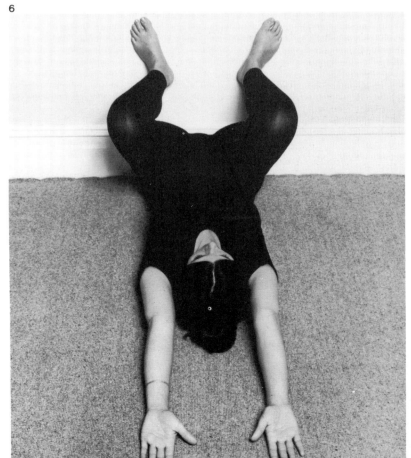

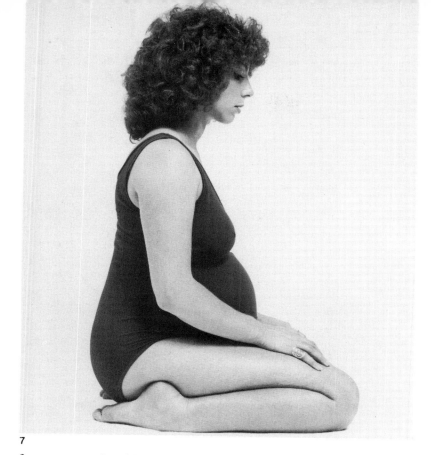

7

from your shoulder bones. Daily practice of this position gradually reduces any stiffness.

How you benefit : in this position your pelvis is tilted upwards and your lower back rounded out. This helps to prevent and relieve lower backache. The vertebrae of your chest and your shoulder joints are extended and opened (your chest is also expanded). Daily practice of this position increases the flexibility of your joints, especially your shoulder joints, and makes your pectoral muscles more elastic and relaxable.

Time : start at about two minutes, gradually increasing to five minutes. Set time daily, undisturbed.

Exercise 7: Sitting between your feet with knees apart

Sit on your heels. Now, taking your feet to the sides, sit on the floor (7). If this is difficult try sitting on a cushion. Make sure your toes turn slightly inwards and your heels outwards. Stiffness in your ankles and knees will make this position difficult. If it is easy for you, your muscles governing the joints are fully relaxable.

How you benefit : this position extends the front of your ankle joint and makes the muscles fully relaxable.

Time : begin with half a minute and increase your time gradually, until you can eventually sit in it for five minutes with ease and comfort. Set time daily, undisturbed.

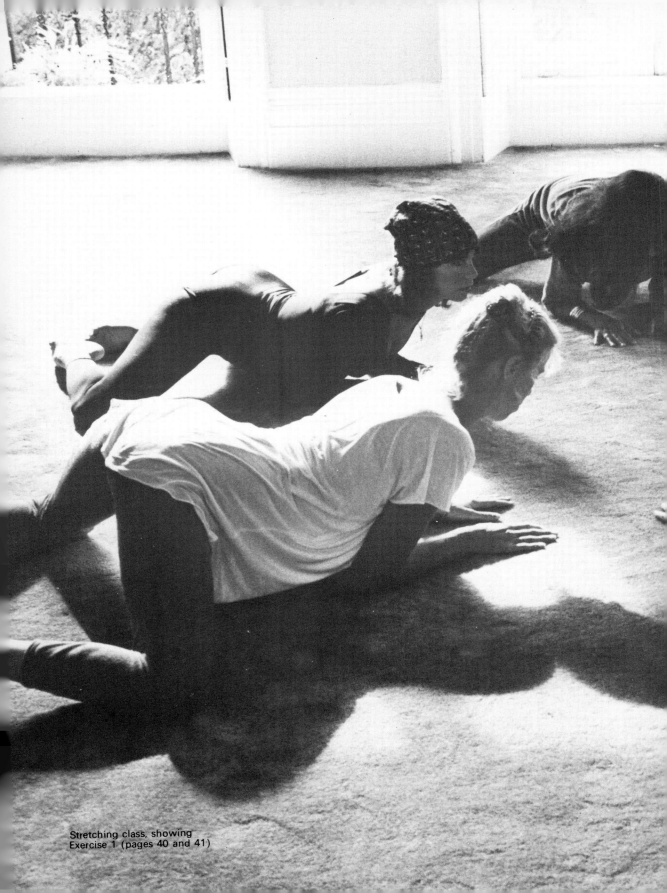

Stretching class, showing
Exercise 1 (pages 40 and 41)

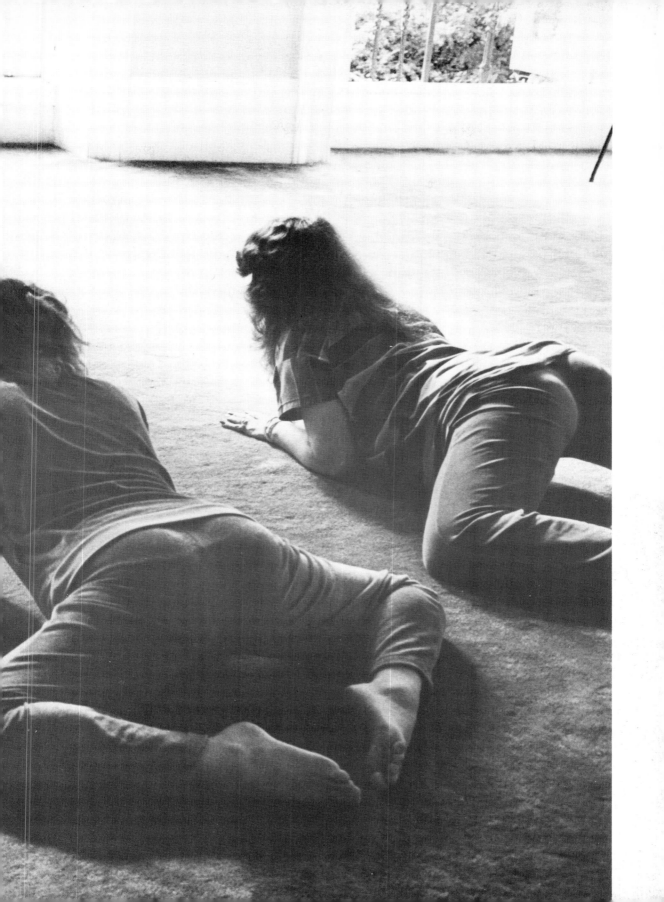

Exercise 8: Twisting

Lie on your back with knees straight and together. Interlock your fingers and place your palms under your head. Bend your knees and bring your feet as close to your buttocks as possible. Now, keeping your elbows on the floor, take both knees to the side (**8a**). Hold this for half a minute then repeat on the other side. Make sure your elbows remain on the floor. If this is difficult, ask someone to hold them gently on to the floor. If it is easy, try the variation with your legs crossed and foot tucked in behind the other leg (**8b**).

How you benefit : this position rotates your spinal column and sacroiliac joints. It is aided by gravity and stretches and relaxes all the oblique muscles of your trunk, your chest, abdomen, and pelvis.

Time : starting with half a minute each side build up to two minutes each side. Set time daily, undisturbed.

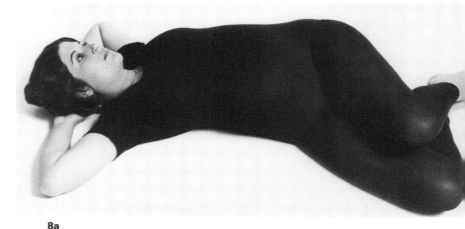

8a

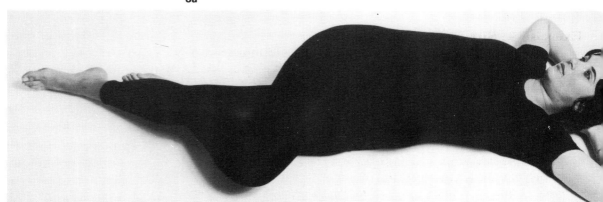

8b

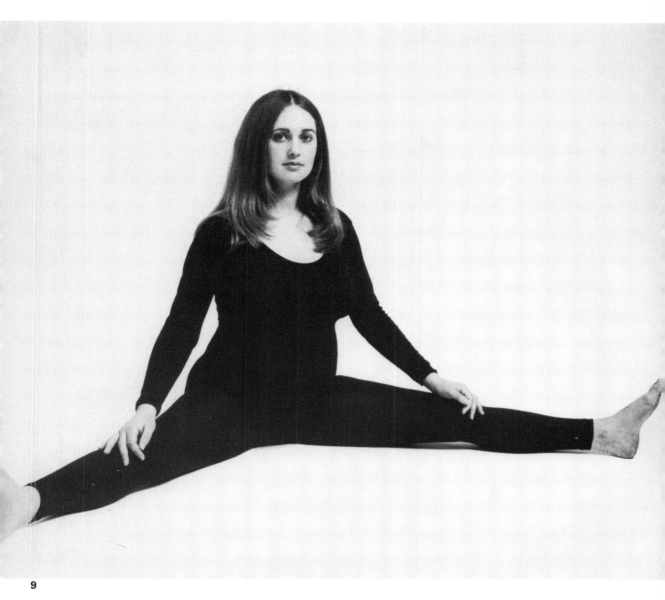

9

Exercise 9 : Sitting with your legs apart

Sit on the floor with your legs close together and extended in front of you. Now spread them apart as far as possible. Make sure your knees are fully extended. Bring your feet slightly towards your knees, extending your heels. Sit upright, trunk straight, with the weight on the front of your buttock bones (**9**). If this is difficult, use a cushion or push backwards with your palms on the floor to lift your buttocks slightly.

How you benefit : this position makes your inner thigh and deep pelvic muscles more relaxable.

Time : begin with half a minute and build up to five minutes. Set time daily, undisturbed.

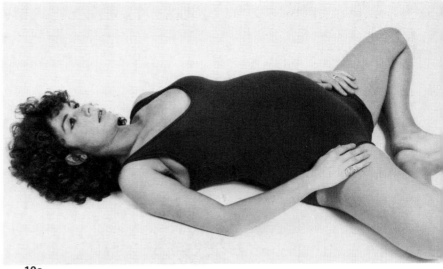

10a

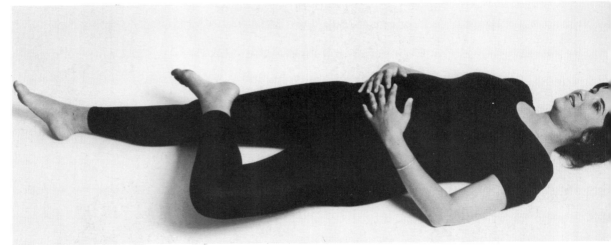

10b

Exercise 10: Tailor position lying on your back
Lie on your back with knees straight. Now bend them and at
the same time bring the soles of your feet together and as close
to your groin as possible. Widen your thighs and allow your
knees to go towards the floor (**10a**).

   As a variation, lie on your back with knees straight. Now
bend one knee and bring your ankle to rest just above your
straightened knee joint. Spread the thigh of your bent knee and
take it towards the floor (**10b**). Repeat with the other leg.

   How you benefit: this position and its variation make the
articular muscles of your hip joints more relaxable.

   Time: begin with the basic position for one minute, building
up to five minutes. For the variation start with a quarter of a
minute each side and build up to two minutes.

Exercise 11: Bending forward from a standing position

Stand with your feet about two feet apart. Hold your left wrist with your right hand, or your right wrist with your left hand, behind you. Bend forward with your hands joined on your buttocks (**11a**). Lever your pelvis and trunk from as far back as possible. Keep your body, from your buttock bones to your head, as straight and easy as possible. Do not bend your neck.

Now lift your shoulder-blades lightly towards your hands. This prevents any strain on your sacroiliac and lower back joints. Use the weight of your trunk as a lever to lengthen the back muscles of your thighs, especially where they meet your lower legs, behind your knees. This is a safe position during pregnancy as long as you remember to bend from your hip joints and not from your back. The simplest way to ensure this is by gently lifting your shoulders towards your hands; just allow your trunk to hang forward without using any effort. If this position is easy for you, try placing your palms on the floor (**11b**).

How you benefit : the weight of your trunk, aided by the force of gravity, stretches, opens, and relaxes your pelvic floor and the backs of your thighs. These thigh muscles are the hamstrings and cultivation of this position reduces their stiffness.

Time : begin with half a minute and increase to five minutes. Set time daily, undisturbed.

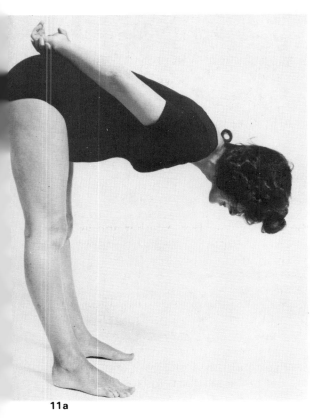

11a

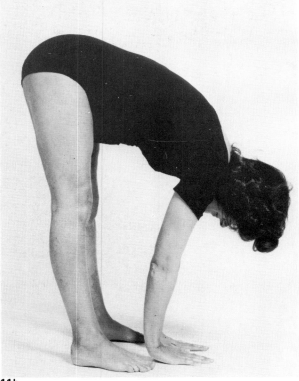

11b

Exercise 12 : Pelvic uptilt

This exercise can be done in several ways. **1** Lie comfortably on your back on the floor, with knees bent and feet on the floor. Now bring your pubic bones towards your breastbone (**12a**). This rounds out your lower back, the small of your back pressing against the floor. Notice how your buttock and abdominal muscles are contracting and closing. Hold this for a few seconds and release. Repeat several times. Then, by pressing down on your heels, tightening your buttock muscles·and lifting your pelvis up off the ground, raise your pubic bone up towards the ceiling and hold for a few seconds, then lower your pelvis gently back onto the ground. Rest for a few seconds and then repeat the whole movement. Do this four or five times.

2 The squatting position, described on page 72, automatically tilts your pelvis up and you don't need to will it. When squatting, unlike the above position, your buttocks and abdominal muscles are not tightening and closing but stretching and opening. By cultivating the pelvic uptilt movement and the squatting position, you are encouraging your buttock and abdominal muscles to be capable of fully opening and fully closing.

3 The all-fours position, with your trunk horizontal and your arms and thighs vertical, is also a very useful position for

12a

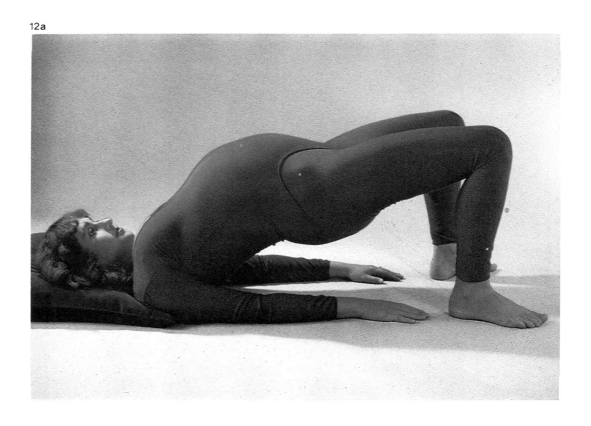

doing the pelvic uptilt and helps to prevent or relieve backache (**12b**).

How you benefit: this exercise is against gravity, and your buttock and inner abdominal muscles (lumbar–iliac) contract against resistance. The aim is to increase the capacity of these muscles to contract, shorten, and close, and so resist weight or force. Your buttock muscles, the largest skeletal muscle group in your body, are, along with your pelvic floor muscles, the guardian muscles of your pelvic outlet. Their efficient contraction and closing ensures good pelvic support for the extra weight of your child during pregnancy, and their full stretchability and opening ensures good pelvic expansion in childbirth.

Time: Begin with ten movements, each of two seconds duration, and build up to ten movements each of five seconds duration. The best way to time seconds is to count out, one thousand and *one*, one thousand and two, one thousand and three, and so on. After months of doing this exercise you will become well aware of the movement of your lower back and the proper tilt when upright. You will automatically hold your pelvis in the best position for support of your abdomen. Slight tightening of your buttock muscles becomes a natural part of your standing position. Movements will become lighter and more graceful, as your lower-back curve is lessened and improved.

12b

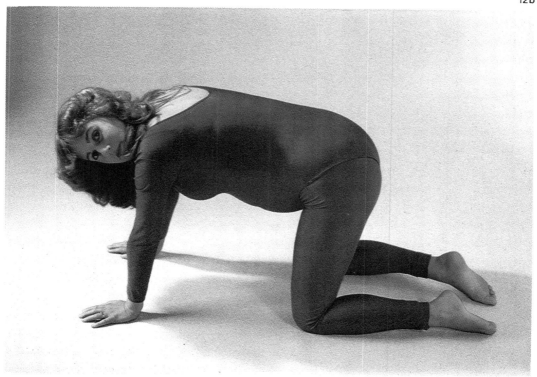

Exercise 13: Alternate closing and resting of your pelvic floor

The muscles of your pelvic floor form a hammock across the bony outlet of your pelvis (see diagram on page 29). They support your bladder, uterus, and rectum and are divided in the centre to allow your urethra (bladder outlet), vagina (uterine outlet) and anus (bowel outlet) to pass through. Unwittingly, every time you try to control a full bladder or rectum, you close and lift your pelvic floor. The muscles are drawn closer together and the whole sling of muscle is lifted and tightened.

Squat on your toes, leaning forward with your hands on the ground, or hold onto a support (see pages 71–73).

1 Close and draw up your anal outlet as if controlling your bowel for a few seconds and rest again. Do this five times. This willed movement is accompanied by a feeling of tightening towards the back of your pelvic floor as your anus is lifted and squeezed.

2 Now close and draw up your vaginal and urethral outlet as if to control your bladder, then rest. Do this five times. This willed movement is accompanied by a feeling of tightening towards the front of your pelvic floor.

3 Close and draw up both your anal and urogenital outlets for a few seconds, then rest. Do this five times. You should sense a definite lift of the whole of your pelvic floor and when you let go you should feel it slacken and descend.

To begin with the sensations of these two movements may seem very much the same, but with time and practice they can easily be differentiated.

These three movements can be done in any position, lying, sitting, standing, squatting, and so on. They can also be combined with the pelvic uptilt movement (**12**).

Summary

Many of these exercises can be done any time. Most women don't do exercises because they think that they have no spare time. The pelvic floor exercises and most of the sitting positions can be built into your daily routine. Doing them can become a pleasant habit.

7 Breathing

The functions of breathing

You breathe to provide the cells of your body with the oxygen they need and to expel the unwanted carbon dioxide. Two operations are involved, internal breathing and external breathing.

Internal breathing involves the delivery by your heart through the bloodstream of the oxygen from your lungs. It is an operation of which you are not physically aware.

External breathing you are aware of. This is the movement of breathing-in and breathing-out, inhaling and exhaling. It involves your entire trunk, which is made up of two cavities. The upper cavity is your chest and the lower your abdomen. They are separated by the sheet of muscle and tendon known as the diaphragm.

The muscles mainly responsible for the rhythmical bellows-like movement of breathing are the diaphragm and the inter-costal muscles, which lie between your ribs. When your

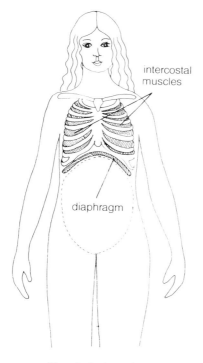

intercostal
muscles

diaphragm

The principal muscles
of breathing

diaphragm contracts, the capacity of your chest cavity is increased from top to bottom. When your intercostal muscles contract your chest cavity is increased from side to side and from back to front.

Try this: place your hands on your ribs, just under your breasts. Then exert a slight pressure as you exhale. Maintain the pressure and keep breathing. You will notice that you are breathing mostly with your diaphragm, causing movement of your abdominal wall. This is abdominal breathing. Now place your hands on your abdomen as you exhale. Now you feel that your chest and collar-bone areas are the most active (and so your intercostal muscles). This is chest breathing.

The breathing cycle

The normal cycle of the breath consists of three phases. *The inhalation* is when the chest expands and the lungs are filled with fresh air. *The exhalation*, during which the elastic chest wall recoils and the stale air is exhaled and the lungs emptied. Between the inhalation and the exhalation there is a third phase, *the retention*, which is a pause after the lungs have emptied and before fresh air is taken in. When we become anxious we tend to inhale forcefully and exhale rapidly, miss the pause altogether, and inhale again before we have completely emptied our lungs of stale air.

If you observe the breathing of a baby or young child you will notice that the belly moves up and down with each inhalation and exhalation. This is abdominal or deep breathing and is the way that nature intended us to breathe. By the time we reach adulthood the stresses and strains of modern life have often taken their toll on our breathing pattern. This usually results in our breathing being restricted to a more shallow chest breathing. The rate of breathing becomes faster than it should be and generally our respiratory system is not functioning at its best.

'During pregnancy your baby in the womb receives all its oxygen and other requirements through the placenta from your blood. All the waste products no longer needed by your child are also passed out through your circulation. If your breathing is restricted, this in turn affects your circulation and the supply of oxygen and removal of carbon dioxide to and from your uterus. Therefore our first aim is to correct any faulty breathing patterns and to learn how to breathe like a baby again.

By paying careful attention to the three phases of the breathing cycle for ten minutes each day, it is possible to restore the normal pattern of the breath within three or four weeks. The result is better breathing and a general calming and relaxation of body and mind. This is of great benefit to you and your baby during pregnancy and forms the foundation of breathing well during labour.

The value of breathing awareness

Breathing is your most obvious bodily rhythm, your most noticeable musical beat. The heart beat may be more consistent and less changeable, but it is less obvious.

Try this: sit back comfortably and quieten yourself. Be as still as you can be. You are able to keep your body motionless and even stop your breathing for a time. After a while you are forced to breathe again. Let your breathing continue and focus your attention on it for a few moments. Just witness it without interference, keeping everything still except your breathing movement. Notice the continual rising and falling of your chest and abdomen (no matter how small this may be).

This simple exercise should convince you that your breathing rhythm is the most convenient and suitable bodily rhythm on which to focus awareness. Breathing is ideal for centring your attention on your body, taking your mind off other matters, such as what happened at work today or yesterday, and so on. Such awareness temporarily stops mental activities such as thinking, fantasizing, remembering and, especially, worrying. This is a valuable tool to have in labour. It prevents your mind from expecting the worst and from unnecessary speculation.

Awareness of your breathing also stops you from interfering with your breathing patterns during uterine contractions, as you might by unintentionally holding or modifying your breath and being unaware that you were doing so. Instead, you allow your breathing to follow the dictates of your uterine contractions undisturbed. In fact, this non-interference automatically improves your involuntary breathing rhythm during uterine contractions. Altogether it is very valuable in labour.

Breathing exercises

The best time to start your breathing practice is early on in your pregnancy, if not before.

Choose a time of day when you can spend fifteen minutes undisturbed in a quiet place. It takes time and regular attention to cultivate deep breathing awareness. At first you may need to make a conscious effort to follow the simple instructions but after a few weeks of regular practice your breathing will become more relaxed and spontaneous.

The exercises that follow are not breathing 'techniques' but simple ways of rediscovering your natural breathing and increasing your ability to centre your awareness on its rhythms. By focusing your attention on your breathing you are helping to still your mind and relax your body. The exercises can be practised alone or together with a partner who will be with you when you are in labour.

How to sit

The first thing to do is to find a relaxed and comfortable sitting position.

Try this: sit on the floor with your back against a wall, tucking your buttocks as close to the wall as possible, your lower back or sacrum and the top of the shoulder blades touching the wall. With knees bent, pull first one foot in towards your body and then place the other in front of it – knees flat on the floor. If you find this difficult then simply sit with legs crossed.

Distribute your weight evenly between your two buttock bones and lift up from the base of your spine. Relax your shoulders by dropping them. Keep your shoulder blades down and open them away from the spine. Rest your hands on your knees, palms upwards, and allow your arms to hang comfortably at your sides being aware of a slight gap between your arms and your torso, starting at the armpits.

Allow your head to hang forward a little and close your eyes.

Alternatively, *try this:* sit on your heels with knees together and place a cushion between your feet and your buttocks. Sit with your spine straight, lifting up from the sacrum. Drop your shoulders, keeping the shoulder blades down and opening them away from the spine so that your chest is open. Allow your arms to hang comfortably, placing your hands on your lap.

Allow your head to hang forward a little and close your eyes.

Breathing Exercise 1

Once you have found a comfortable sitting position sit quietly for a few moments and direct your attention inwards to the rhythm of your breathing. Allow your whole body to relax and hang comfortably. Drop your shoulders, relax the muscles of your face, allow all tension to melt away until your face feels soft and smooth. Relax your jaw and throat, releasing unnecessary tension and allow yourself to be open and receptive.

Without doing anything at all just become aware of your breathing, the inhalation, the exhalation and the pause in between. Notice which parts of your body are moving when you breathe.

Now try breathing in through your nose and breathing out through your mouth. Each time you breathe out empty your lungs completely, slowly sighing the breath out until there is none left. Then pause for a few seconds until you feel like breathing in. Then draw in a new breath allowing your lungs to fill slowly from the bottom up, rather like water filling a jug.

With each inhalation you are drawing in energy in the form of breath as gently as you draw in the fragrance of a flower. With each exhalation your body discharges the outgoing breath from the top of the chest, slowly releasing to below the navel. The exhalation releases tension and calms and relaxes the body.

Spend a few minutes inhaling and exhaling systematically (in through your nose and out through your mouth) and pay close attention to the rhythm and pattern of the breath. Concentrate on the exhalation and remember the pause between each breath.

Return to your normal breathing in and out through the nose. Keep your attention focused on the breath, your eyes closed and body relaxed. When thoughts arise try not to focus on them but simply let them go. Witness the rise and fall of your breathing. Continue to meditate quietly in this way for a few minutes and then slowly open your eyes.

Practise Exercise 1 daily for a week or two until it becomes effortless. When you are ready, add the following exercises.

Breathing Exercise 2

Sit comfortably and become aware of your breathing. Breath in through your nose and out through your mouth, pausing between each breath and concentrating on the exhalation. Continue like this for a few minutes and while you are doing so direct your attention to your abdomen, finding a spot a couple of inches below your navel.

Try to lower your breathing so that each time you inhale you are breathing towards this spot and each time you exhale you are breathing away from this spot.

It should feel as if your belly fills with air when you breathe in and empties each time you breathe out.

Place your hands on your lower belly and continue to breathe in this way. Feel your belly rising gently towards your hands with each inhalation and falling way from your hands with each exhalation as if emptying. It's as if your belly expands and comes out when you breath in and withdraws and goes in when you breathe out.

You may find this a little difficult at first, particularly if you have become used to breathing more shallowly into your chest. However, by making a conscious effort to breathe abdominally, after a few weeks you will be able to do it spontaneously – like a baby! With regular practice your breathing will deepen and become slower and more efficient, your concentration will increase and you will begin to feel calm and relaxed.

After breathing into your belly for a few minutes place your hands on your knees, palms up, and return to your normal breathing, in and out through the nose, before finishing the exercise.

Practice breathing deeply into your belly when you do your stretching exercises and allow yourself to breathe away the tension in your body. This is very good practice for breathing through contractions in labour.

Breathing Exercise 3

Kneel forward onto your hands and knees with your knees slightly apart. Rotate your hips in a circle as if you were in the middle of a strong contraction in labour.

Breathe deeply in through the nose and out through the

mouth. Concentrate on the outbreath and imagine that you are breathing through the contraction. Continue, rotating your hips in the opposite direction.

Try practising this breathing exercise in different birth positions, such as standing and leaning foward onto a wall, sitting or squatting. You may find it helpful practising this with a partner, breathing together and including some massage of the lower back so that your movements, the massage and your breathing all work together in harmony.

Breathing Exercise 4

Squat down on your toes and lean forward using your hands to support your body. Close your eyes and focus your attention inwards on the rhythm of your breathing. Breathe in through the nose and out slowly through the mouth, pausing in between breaths. Let your awareness centre on your pelvic floor and with each exhalation release your pelvic floor muscles.

Imagine that your baby's head (about the size of a grapefruit) is descending during the second stage of labour. With each exhalation imagine the head coming lower and all the soft tissues of the vagina and pelvic floor releasing and opening to allow the baby to be born. Imagine that you could 'breathe your baby out'. When you are in labour your uterus will contract strongly from above to push your baby out. You may want to go along with these powerful expulsive efforts and work with the contractions, bearing down when you feel the urge, or you may find it more helpful to just relax, let go, and breathe your baby out slowly while your uterus does all the work.

You may want to breathe quietly or to let out a lot of sound as you breathe out, it doesn't matter so long as you breathe out and do not hold your breath. Several small 'pushes' work just as well as one long one. Try this exercise in other second stage positions such as standing or kneeling.

Breathing Exercise 5

Squat down on your toes and lean forward using your hands to support your body. Imagine that your baby's head is 'crowning' and that you are just on the brink of actually giving birth.

Breathe deeply and slowly, concentrating on the exhalation. Imagine your uterus contracting and that you are feeling a very powerful urge to bear down. Pant lightly as the urge is at its strongest and then go back to breathing deeply as it begins to wear off and your baby's head comes through. By breathing in this way at the moment of birth you allow the perineal tissues time to release and this can help to avoid a tear. However, some women prefer not to use conscious control at this point and just let go. Many women spontaneously cry out as their child emerges and there is a 'primal' birth cry which sounds very similar in all women regardless of which culture they come from or language they speak.

Breathing for labour

Once you have practised Exercises 1 to 5 regularly you are ready for labour. You do not need any 'breathing techniques' to see you through the contractions as you have cultivated the art of awareness and concentration on the breath. There is no need to pay any special attention to the contractions until they become so strong that you need to concentrate on them. Then, as you feel the contraction coming on, simply breathe deeply into your abdomen, concentrating on the outbreath. Make sure that you are in a comfortable position so that you can relax completely and let go of your whole body, breathing your way over the peak and through the contraction. In this way you go deeper 'into' the contraction, rather than trying to distract yourself away from it. Combined with a sensible upright position this sort of breathing will help you to stay calm and relaxed and will help to release anxiety, tension and pain.

Deep breathing will help you to sink deeply inwards during the labour. It will help you to allow yourself to be open and to accept the change of consciousness involved in giving birth. It will help you to let go of inhibitions and fears – to get in touch with the primitive instincts you have within your body and to trust your own potentials.

During the labour you may discover your own kind of breathing – you may breathe quietly or you may make a lot of noise, or sing, moan or hum. By starting off with deep breathing, you can allow yourself to discover your own way of breathing through the contractions.

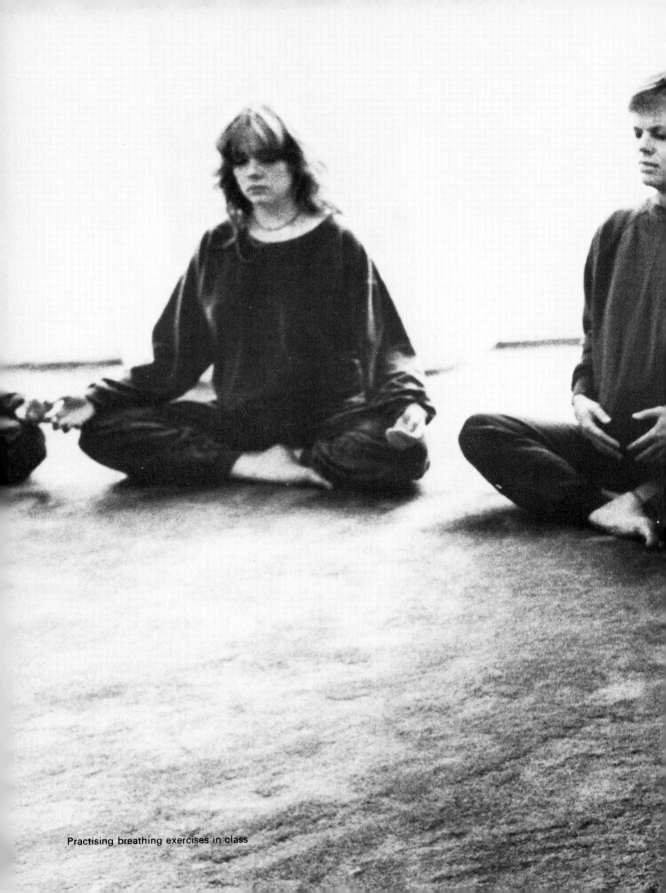

Practising breathing exercises in class

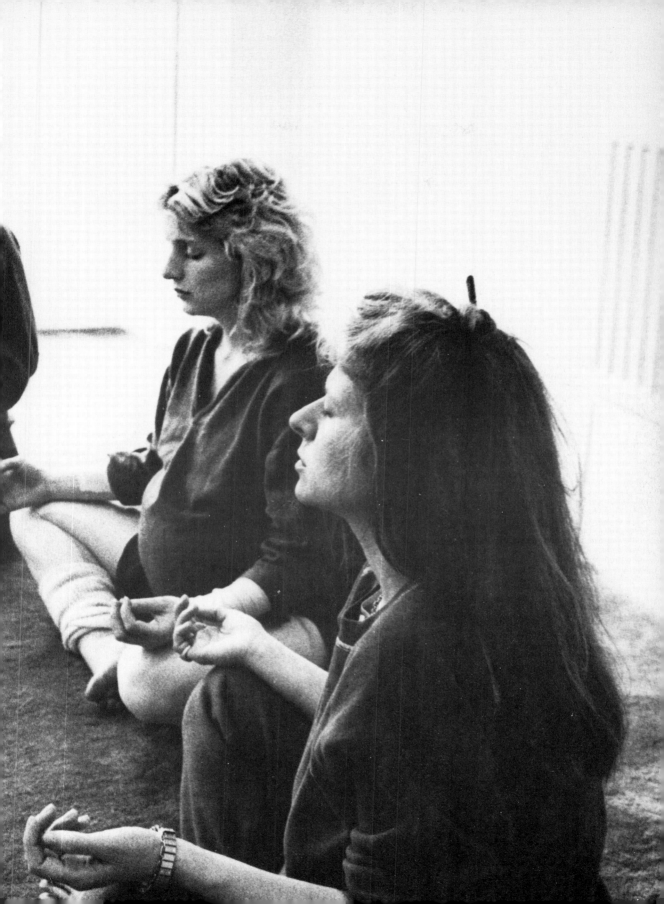

8 Squatting

Exercise 1

Although many positions are suitable for labour and delivery (otherwise birth would not take place in them) some are more so than others. Seven positions are most effective.

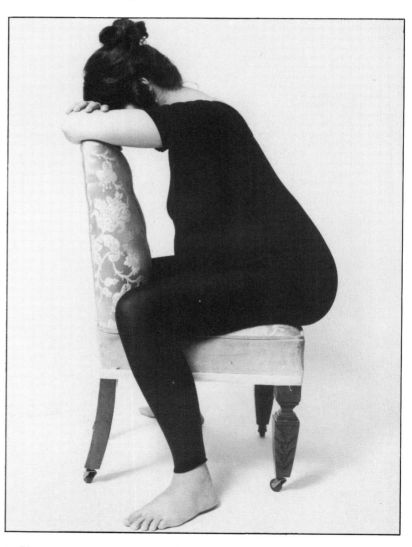

1 Sitting on a chair reversed around so that you rest your trunk on its backrest. (This position may be used mainly during contractions in the first stage of labour.)

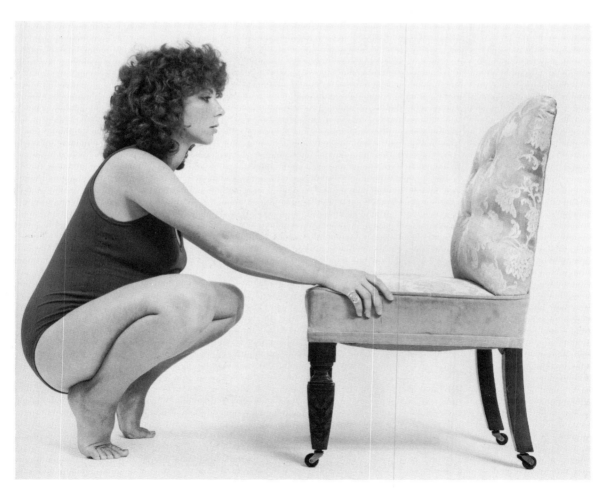

2 The squatting position, on your toes with knees comfortably
apart and supporting yourself with the chair.

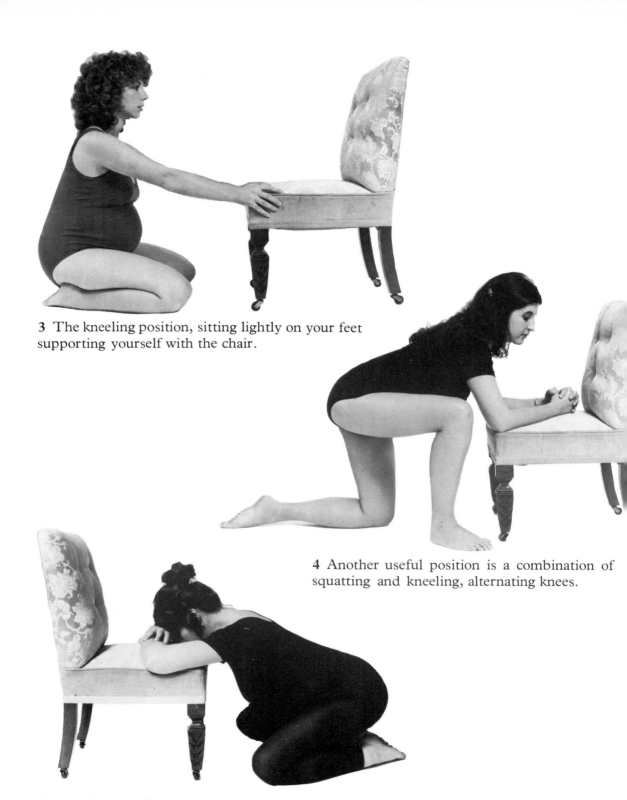

3 The kneeling position, sitting lightly on your feet supporting yourself with the chair.

4 Another useful position is a combination of squatting and kneeling, alternating knees.

5 A similar kneeling position, but leaning forward and resting on your head and arms.

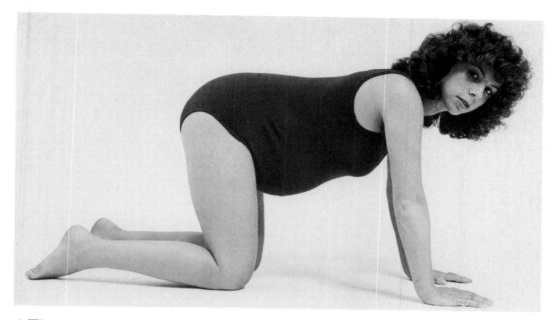

6 The all-fours position, with your back slightly bent and rounded.

7 The knee-chest position, resting your head and upper trunk on a mat or cushion on the floor, or on a low bed.

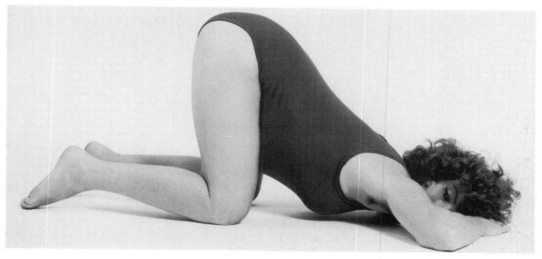

Begin practising the seven positions by sitting on a reversed chair, then squat, and so on all the way through to the knee-chest position (**1**). These positions should, with practice, become easily changeable at a moment's notice.

Every woman will vary in her ability to carry out the positions, but should cultivate them gradually. Stay in a position only as long as you find it relatively comfortable. To go on longer is to miss the point. These are not lessons in sheer effort, but in how gradually to turn difficult positions into easy ones.

Exercise 2: Squatting

You may have most difficulty with the exercise of squatting even though as a child you instinctively squatted when you first began to crawl, stand, and walk. If you cannot squat now you have lost the ability you once had. This may be because of stiff ankle joints and stiff, shortened achilles tendons and calf-muscles. It is easier to squat with heeled shoes or on your toes as this does not demand the full stretch and relaxation of these muscles. There may be stiffness in the extensor muscles of your knees and/or in the muscles of your groin. When you first begin to squat, you may experience pain or aching in your ankles or knees or groin. With practice these soon disappear.

There are two ways to squat: one with heels on the floor, which is a resting position; the other on your toes, which is an expulsive position (**1**). On your toes is easier, but you can't stay in it for long without support. With support, it is most suitable for the expulsive stage of labour. If you can comfortably squat on your heels, squatting on your toes can be taken for granted. The following exercise therefore centres on the more difficult position of squatting with heels flat on the floor.

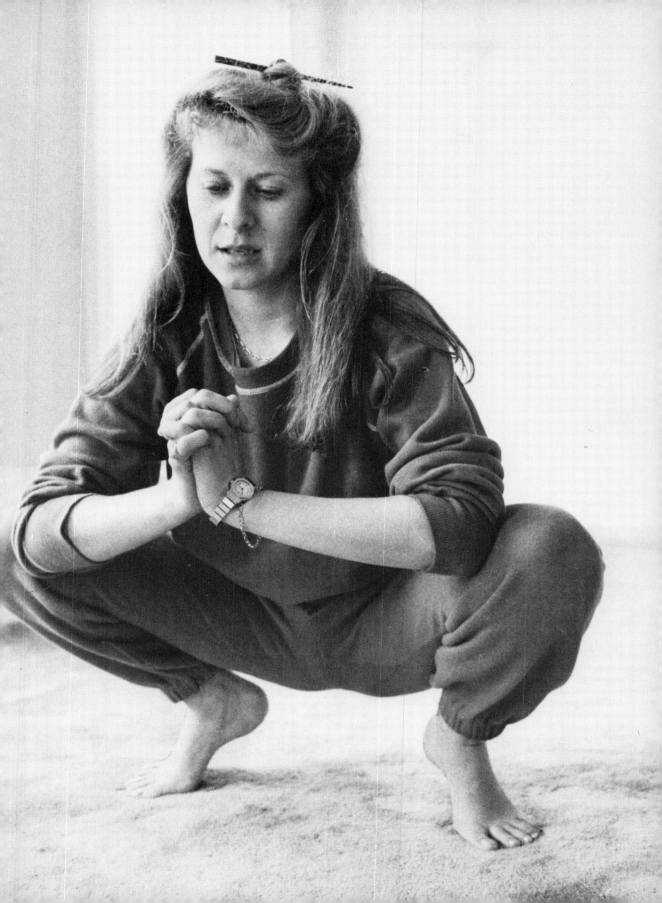

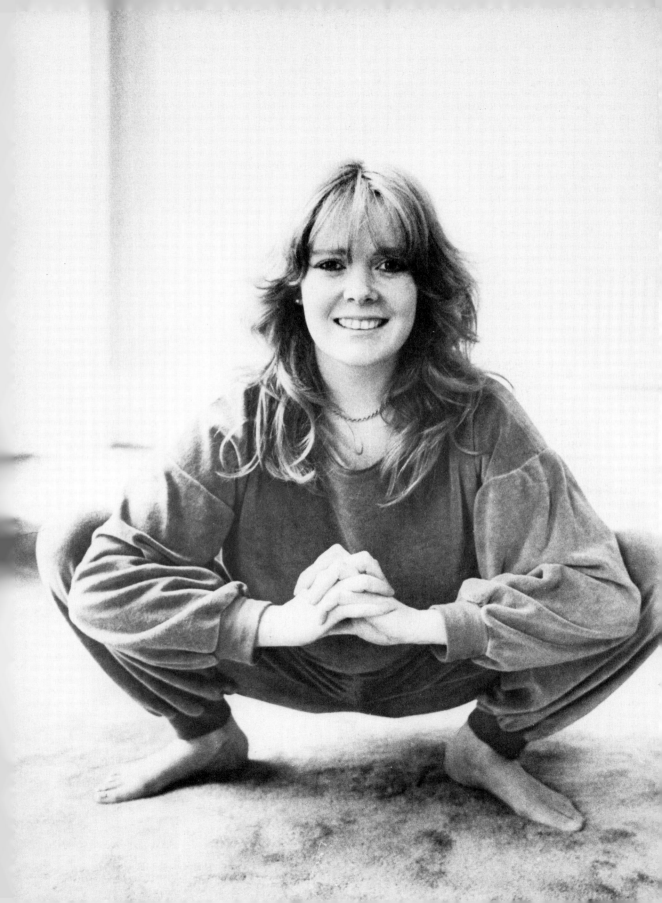

Squatting without support : stand with your feet about eighteen inches apart, toes turned outwards. Now bend your knees and squat, keeping your knees comfortably apart and your heels flat on the floor (**2a**). Rest in this position for a minute or so and come up again by pressing your feet on the floor and straightening your knees and hips.

If you can do this, your task is then to build up your ease and time in this position through the months of pregnancy. Begin at a minute, say ten times a day; then two minutes five times a day; then five minutes twice a day, and finally ten minutes twice a day. Devise your own time schedule until you can with relative ease squat for five minutes at a time.

Squatting in supported positions : if you cannot squat unaided, or if you fall over or are forced to lift your heels and go onto your toes or find it painful, your joints and muscles are stiff, so begin with the following supported positions.

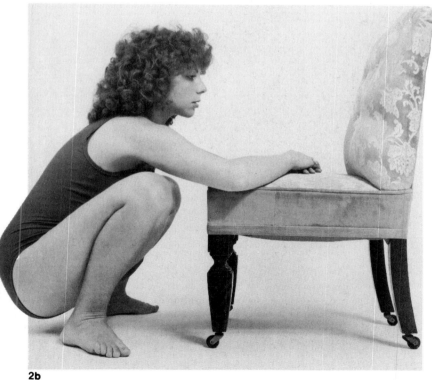

2b

Find something that can support the full weight of your body, the end of a heavy table or bed or a strong door handle. Hold on to it and, with your feet about eighteen inches apart and turning slightly outwards, bend your knees and gradually go into a squatting position (**2b**). Keep your heels flat on the floor and your knees comfortably apart. Stay in the position for a minute or so. Come up again by pressing your feet on the floor and straightening your knees and hips.

Or stand with your back to a wall with your feet about six inches in front of the wall and about eighteen inches apart from each other. Leaning against the wall, slide your back gently down (**2c**). Rest in this position for a minute or so and come up.

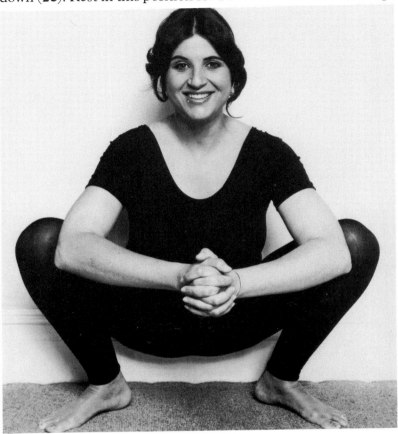

2c

Whichever supported position you choose, begin at half a minute and then gradually increase this to five minutes at a time. When this is easy, go on to the next stage without support.

Daily practice of squatting over several months, ten minutes a day, helps to prevent and relieve backache, constipation, varicose veins, and muscle cramps, besides making your joints more flexible and your muscles more relaxable. Squatting is one of the most sensible positions for labour and delivery.

Inclining and reclining positions

Any position in which it is possible for birth to take place must be suitable to some degree. Therefore the issue about labour and delivery positions is which are more suitable and why. They may be divided into two groups; reclining positions and inclining positions. In the reclining group you lie down, with the back or side of your trunk resting on something so that you are backwards from the vertical or upright position.

In inclining positions you stoop or bend your trunk forwards from the upright position.

The almost universal conventional positions currently used for delivery are:

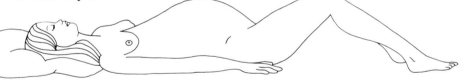

1 *the dorsal*, in which you lie flat on your back with knees up and separated;

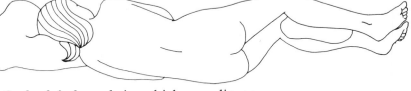

2 *the left lateral*, in which you lie on your left side, knees towards your chest;

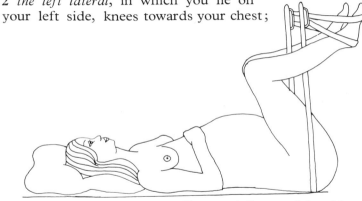

3 *the lithotomy position*, usually on a delivery table with stirrups (this is the one normally used in the United States);

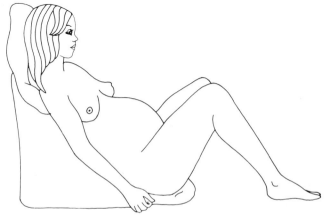

4 *the semi-upright position*, supported by cushions (the usual position adopted in Britain).

These are all reclining positions. Why do modern obstetrics seem to demand that you give birth reclining when historical and medical evidence as well as natural instinct and common sense, support inclining positions?

Historical evidence

There is evidence going back thousands of years of the bodily positions taken in childbirth. The head of a silver pin from Luristan in Iran, first millennium BC, depicts a squatting mother. The remains of a clay statue from the ruins of Satal Huyak, a Stone Age city of about 7000 to 5000 BC in Turkey, shows a woman giving birth in the same position. An eight-and-a-half-inch Aztec fertility stone figure from Mexico depicts giving birth squatting. A relic of the Mound Builders of Eastern Arkansas, a pre-Columbian culture of unknown date, shows a woman squatting with her hands on her thighs. Egyptian hieroglyphs meaning 'to give birth' show a mother squatting.

A relief from the Temple of Esna, a town on the Nile in Upper Egypt, shows a princess giving birth in the kneeling position. Birth in the same position can be seen in a marble figure from Sparta, about 500 BC. In Ancient China and Japan, women customarily gave birth in the kneeling position on a straw mat. All scenes, of course, depict only the final birth, but positions used during the rest of labour can also be traced.

Exodus, chapter 1, verse 16, states: 'When ye do the office of a midwife, go to the Hebrew women and see them upon *the stools*'. A Corinthian vase depicts a woman in labour seated on a birth chair. An early Greek relief and a Roman marble bas-relief both show a woman giving birth on a stool supported by two assistants.

The birthstool was recommended for uncomplicated labours by Soranus in the early second century AD and by many subsequent writers. It was described as 'in form like a barber's chair but with a crescent-shaped opening in the seat, through which the child may fall'. The first birthstools must have been rocks or logs of wood, developing over time into complex, adjustable chairs with many varied devices.

From birthchair to bed and delivery table

In the Western world the birthstool or chair remained indispensably part of the equipment of most midwives up to the middle of the eighteenth century. Each wealthy household had its own stool, while among the poor, a stool was transported from house to house. The birthstools of royalty were carved and ornamented with jewels. Dutch, German and French sixteenth-century drawings show the great use of the birthstool, as do Chinese drawings of the same period. Even today a birthchair is still used by some Egyptian women.

François Mauriceau, the leading figure in French obstetrics of the seventeenth century, scorned the use of the birthchair and advocated childbirth in bed. As forceps gained popularity, the birthchair lost favour and by the end of the eighteenth century little more was heard of it. The birthchair gave way to the bed and the delivery tables of the nineteenth and twentieth centuries. Women were now flat on their backs, a position that offered a fine view to the attendant but was in total defiance of the active forces of gravity and of the independence that comes from giving birth on one's own two feet. Nor did this position encourage the labouring woman to utilize her own efforts.

Primitive women

Primitive tribes have adopted various birth positions through customs of their tribe, but more important, by their instinct. Some forty positions have been recorded, and their relative merits have been much disputed. Women of different tribes squat, kneel, stand, incline, sit or lie on the belly; so, too, do they vary their positions in various stages of labour and difficult labours.

Dr G. J. Englemann, in his book *Labour Among Primitive Peoples* written in 1883, was one of the first to investigate the various positions assumed in labour and childbirth by different peoples, and he found that the four principal positions were squatting, kneeling (including the all-fours and knee-chest positions), standing and recumbent.

The custom of animals

Most four-legged animals give birth on all-fours or on their sides; squatting is not a resting position for them. Those that do give birth on their sides often extend their front legs so that the head and upper trunk is upright. They need their mouths to chew through the umbilical cord and to clean their young. Also they effect a little leverage with their front or back legs or both, against the ground or any obstacle that happens to be close by. Lying on their sides secures an immediate place of rest close to the maternal opening for the newborn young.

Animals that are able to squat and have the use of their front limbs (hands), monkeys, apes, gorillas, and so on, mostly give birth squatting.

Safety

What are the basic conditions that make a position suitable for childbirth?

The first essential is that the position must be safe for you and your child. When joints, which are the roots of bodily positions and movements, are flexed (closed) they are more stable and protected from injury than when they are extended (opened). When your child is in the foetal position within you, most of its joints are flexed (closed) because of the compact space and because they are thus in their safest positions.

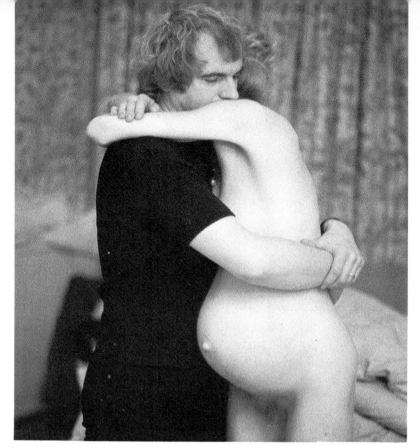

This sequence of photographs shows an active birth (standing) in a hospital delivery room

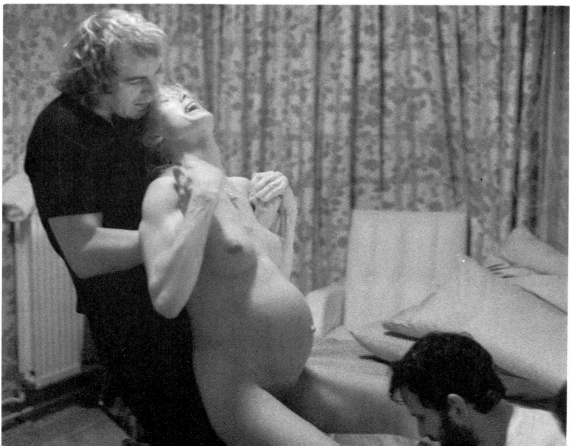

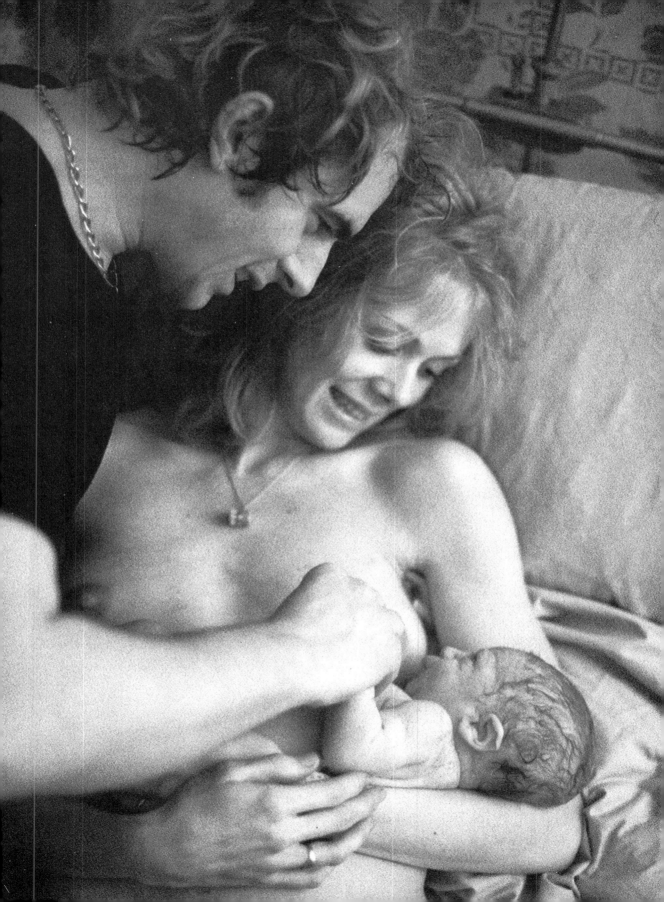

In the standing position the pelvis is tilted slightly forward

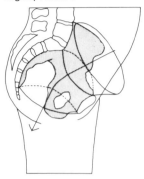

In the reclining position the pelvis is positioned on its back, so that the child going through it must go upwards against the force of gravity, which demands more effort from the uterus

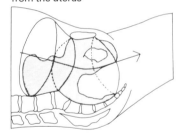

In the squatting position and other inclining positions the pelvis is almost vertical and the descending child takes the line of least resistance

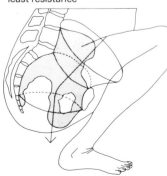

For you, in the expulsive effort of childbirth, a position is safe when it promotes the closing of your abdomen and the opening of your pelvis. When you are squatting, most of your bodily joints are flexed and closed except those of your pelvis, which are opened. So your pelvis is at its widest and the rest of your trunk at its narrowest or smallest. This aids the expulsion of your child. Your pelvis is tilted upwards and your lower back vertebrae rounded out and flexed, which are their least vulnerable and strained positions. As a result, squatting is the safest position of childbirth and kneeling is the next safest. On the other hand, any position that extends your back, thighs, and knees and that opens your abdomen and closes your pelvis is unsuitable and unsafe.

Resting

The second essential that makes a position suitable for childbirth is that it places your body in a resting or relaxing position. Your body must be freed from the task of supporting itself so that energy may be made available for the expulsive actions of your uterus and should not be wasted on supporting your body.

Lying on your back or side is a resting position, your muscles are inactive. But, as we have already seen, muscles can be inactive in terms of energy but mechanically active, some of them are shortening (closing) and others are stretching (opening), a more dynamic state of relaxation. Squatting and kneeling are mechanically active resting (relaxing) positions, whereas lying on your back or side are mechanically inactive resting positions.

There is no doubt that your bodily position affects your attitude. So when squatting or kneeling, while you are relaxed you are also mechanically active, self-reliant and in a position of preparedness. Lying down, on the other hand, makes you feel passive and helpless.

You do not choose to lie on your back or on your side to pass urine or to evacuate your bowels. You do so uncomfortably, only when you are ill. Childbirth is also an expulsive action, so it is logical and instinctive for a woman in labour to adopt crouching or inclining positions in preference to reclining ones; it is absurd to reject the invaluable help that gravity offers you.

Try this : lie on your back on the floor, lift your head for a few seconds to experience your abdominal muscles tightening and with your hands feel their definition and hardness. Do not hold this position too long as these muscles are straining. The mere lifting of your head hardens these muscles.

Now squat, using a support, and feel with your hands these same muscles. They feel much softer. Yet they are shortening to their maximum with the assistance of gravity and without effort or tightening. If you lie down to give birth, each movement of your head and trunk hardens and strains these muscles; they are working against gravity. Also, in the expulsive stage of labour they often contract involuntarily to aid your uterus. If you are squatting or kneeling this happens with ease as they are assisted by gravity, whereas when lying on your back, effort and strain are needed.

The all-fours position is a horizontal resting position, in which the trunk of your body makes no contact with the floor.

Leverage
The third essential that makes a position suitable for childbirth is to have something, the floor or any obstacle, to push against. Your pelvis needs to be anchored as your child is pushed out through it by your shrinking uterus. This helps expulsion.

For your uterus to contract and retract sufficiently and economically you need to have force exerted on your pelvis in the opposite direction to that of your uterus. This is so because your uterine muscles when contracting pull against your pelvis to which they are attached (see diagram).

Four-legged animals effect slight leverage with their front or back legs, or both (at moments of exceptional exertion) against any obstacle that happens to be close by. A cat or a bitch usually uses the sides of its basket for this. For a woman, when squatting and kneeling, the floor provides the resistance; no supports are needed. On the other hand, most beds do not offer supports or points of resistance by means of which you can assist yourself at the critical moments. This is another disadvantage in lying in bed on your back or side. Whatever happens, in the second stage of labour don't allow yourself to toss about on a bed which offers you little firm support.

There are other objections to giving birth lying on a bed. The tail-end of your spinal column, the lower sacrum and coccyx are pushed back by pressure on the inside as your child passes by and this widens the front to back diameter of your pelvic outlet. They spring back into their original positions when the pressure has gone. For this reason lying on your back, unlike any upright inclining position, renders your spinal column useless as a lever for positioning your sacrum and coccyx during the second stage.

Blood flow and strength of contractions
A modern textbook, *The Fundamentals of Obstetrics and Gynaecology*, published in 1969, states that: 'There is evidence that in the supine position [lying on your back] the weight of the contracting uterus reduces the placental blood flow by compressing the descending aorta [the large artery of your heart] and inferior vena cava [the large veins leading to your heart.' It also says that the strength of uterine contractions diminishes by one-third when you lie on your back.

The vulnerable perineum
When you are reclining during labour, as your child's head comes through your pelvis, its weight falls on the sacral part of your pelvic floor, adding strain and stress to it.

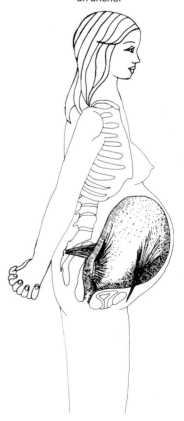

The uterus is attached to the pelvis. When it contracts (pulls) and shrinks, it does so using the pelvis as an anchor

In the squatting, kneeling, and all-fours positions your perineum (the area between your vagina and anus) is not as vulnerable to injury as when reclining. These upright inclining positions take a vertical load off the sacral or anal part of your pelvic floor. This is a crucial consideration.

After taking these facts into consideration, you may realize that labour and childbirth were not meant to take place lying on your back. This is not to say that you should not lie down during labour, but that it should never be the dominant position of a healthy woman.

False arguments

Many authorities on childbirth agree that inclining positions, kneeling and sitting are superior to lying on your back or side or to reclining back on cushions in a semi-upright position (often known as the modified squatting position). 'Sure,' they say, 'squatting or kneeling are better theoretically, but they are not practical.' They seem to justify this with three basic arguments. Reclining positions, they say, are more convenient for the assistants (the physician and midwife), allow better manual care by an assistant of your perineum in delivery, and that most women find squatting, kneeling, and so on too difficult, unfamiliar, and undignified.

These arguments do not stand up to the dictates of common sense. The only time to stay lying in bed is when machines or drips are attached to your body and a change of positions may disturb these attachments.

Convenient view and accessibility

A good view and easy accessibility for the assistants during birth are undoubtedly necessary in most instances. But they can have both merely by your adopting the all-fours or knee-chest positions each time you need to be examined and in the final stages of delivery when the tissues of your vulnerable perineum may be manually eased by your assistant. Even the use of forceps when necessary may be as convenient on all-fours as when reclining.

The Knee-chest position
In this position gravity resists the movement of the child, thus slowing down its exit

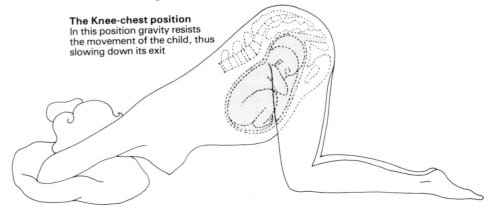

Also, in the all-fours and knee-chest positions you are able to participate and control more. If your child is coming through your vagina too fast and you need to slow down its progress, the all-fours position is ideal as your trunk is horizontal and the force of gravity is reduced. This force may be further diminished and delivery made even slower by adopting the knee-chest position in which your trunk is slightly inverted or upside down (see diagram), plus, as recommended in chapter 7, shallow mouth breathing and light panting.

False delicacy

The false delicacy that prevents many women from assuming the squatting, kneeling, and especially the all-fours and knee-chest positions, can only be ascribed to a refusal to admit that in our vital functions we are still animals. From any rational point of view the all-fours and other inclining positions are no more undignified than the reclining positions, particularly the lithotomy positions in which stirrups are used.

The ability to assume natural positions

For primitive women squatting is the most natural thing in the world. But women in the more highly developed world, who were able to squat comfortably in childhood, often find crouching positions difficult in adulthood. So they compromise and are encouraged to do so. This is a pity because squatting and kneeling are ideal expulsive positions. If you have to strain and feel unsteady, it is certainly not the positions at fault but rather your stiffness. With regular practice during pregnancy, squatting will not be so unfamiliar or difficult by the day of labour.

In fact no single position is 'best' for *all* stages of labour and delivery. In an effort to discover whether there was a natural, instinctive birth position, the obstetrician F. C. Naegele observed a young woman giving birth for the first time. Left alone during labour in a room containing a bed, chair, couch and birthstool, she assumed every possible position on each. Finally she gave birth reclining on the bed.

Some women resist all attempts to get them to go to bed when contractions begin. They insist on giving birth on their hands and knees and do so quite safely.

To be able to move and change your bodily position during labour is a natural, instinctive response that should be open to you. You should feel free to squat, lie, sit, kneel, walk, in fact to assume any comfortable position in which you can assist the task of your uterus and the muscles of the birth canal. This response is not available to you if you are on your back with your legs in stirrups or connected to medical equipment that forces you to be still. But if you insist on having the choice, it is essential that you have seriously cultivated a number of simple, suitable positions during pregnancy so that during labour and childbirth your response will be automatic.

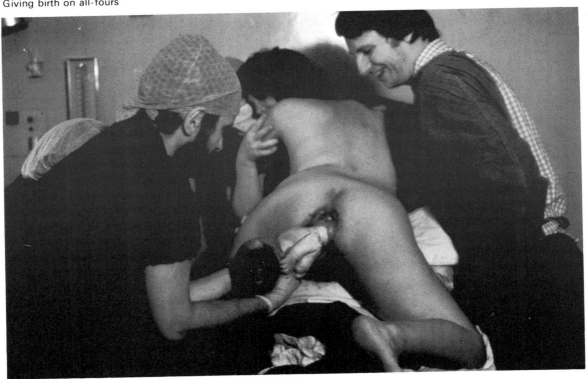

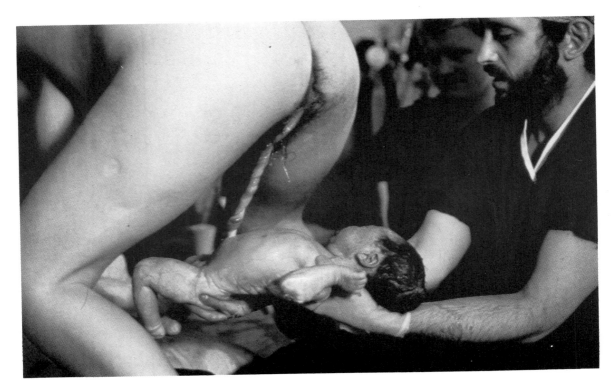

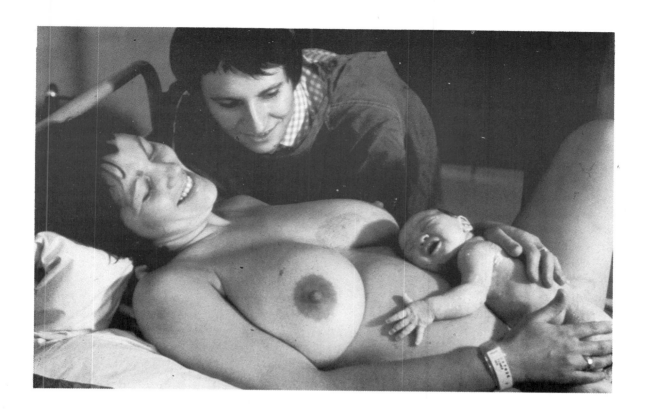

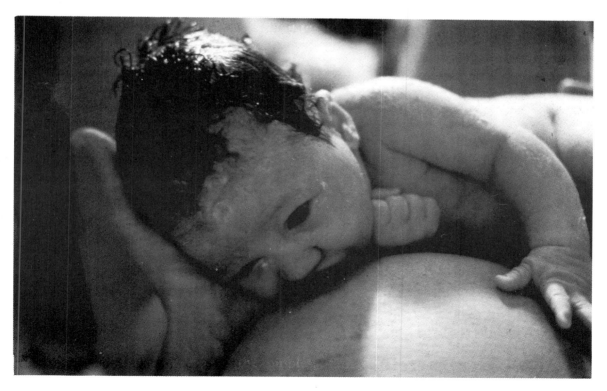

9 Touching and massage

Self-examination and self-massage
You probably know your body most of all from looking at it.
But you can add to that knowledge through your sense of touch.
The tools for this are those remarkable instruments, your hands.

Pregnancy is an appropriate time to examine and massage
your body. The word massage comes from the Portuguese
ammasar, to knead, but as well as kneading, massage involves
stroking, friction, pressure, and other variations of touch. The
aim of massage is stimulation of the soft tissues of your body.
This stimulation can be deep or very light depending on what
is needed. It assists blood circulation and increases the suppleness and relaxation of your tissues.

Apart from such lubricants as oil and ointment, massage is
the only way of directly treating your skin. Such physical
discomforts as tightness, aches, and pains can be alleviated or
lessened and the pleasure is immense. Touching parts of your
body somehow helps, be it an itch, ache, tightening or pain.
It's natural and instinctive.

There is no mystery in massage and if you try it, you will be
surprised at the magic you hold in your hands. With curiosity,
practice and patience you can learn to touch and examine all
parts of your body and develop your own ways of massage.
Almost instinctively you will find how to do this and you will
have the advantage of being able to regulate the pressure you
exert to what you can bear.

Massage made simple
The many textbook movements of massage can be reduced
to four.
1 Surface stroking with the flat of your hand. In severe pain or
spasm this very light stroking is often the only form of massage
possible.
2 Deep stroking, which is done in the same way, but with
greater pressure.
3 Friction, which is carried out by pressing with the tips of
your fingers and thumbs.
4 Kneading, which is done by alternately squeezing and
releasing a muscle.

You can use one or both hands, and any part of your hand
(fingers, thumb, flat, back or sides), provided you exert enough
pressure. Where possible, massage in the direction ·of your
venous flow, towards your heart.

The simplest instruction is to explore and press, probe to find the painful parts and apply friction to dissolve the pain. Once you are good at this, you are then in the position, when massaged by another, to guide them to the parts in need.

Self-massage exercises

The best time for self-massage is after a bath. Take a different part of your body each time. For instance, begin with your feet, then go from your ankles to your knees, next from your knees to your groin, then your abdominal wall and so on until you reach your face and head. For less accessible parts different positions are necessary, but you will soon find the ones that suit you.

Having examined and massaged each section of your body a few times over a period of several weeks or months, you should eventually be able to deal with your entire body in ten to fifteen minutes. Doing this after each bath gives your body the attention and invigoration it deserves, especially during pregnancy.

Abdominal massage

During pregnancy your abdominal muscles, tissues and skin are gradually stretched. The skin may be helped to prepare for this stretching by applying some lubricant such as baby oil, almond oil or liquid lanoline. This nourishes your skin and helps prevent the formation of zig-zag lines and a loose, wrinkled abdomen. The oil or cream should be well massaged into your skin. Again, the best time to do this is after a bath. Begin this from about the fourth month of pregnancy when your uterus has risen out of your pelvis into your abdomen. Your skin may then retain its normal soft elastic texture.

In labour, a soothing self-massage of your lower abdomen during uterine contractions is often very helpful. It needs a very delicate touch and you should practise this after rubbing in the oil. Lightly place your fingertips on your lower belly. Curve the fingers around in an arch from one side of your pubic bone to the other around the shape of your child without completing the circle. Continue this half-circling each time, taking your fingers off before you complete the circle. Do it in rhythm with your out-breath.

Massage by another

There are three kinds of massage which may be very effective during labour and should be practised during pregnancy. These relieve muscle tension, aches, and pains, not only during labour but whenever you feel these physical discomforts in pregnancy.

The first is having your thighs massaged. This is very helpful if you get tightening or cramp there.

The second is having your lower back and pelvis massaged if, during pregnancy or in labour, you experience backache or feel your uterine contractions in your back instead of in your belly or thighs.

The third is the very delicate arch-like touching, during intense contractions. Some women find it more soothing if applied by someone else. It seems to some to take the edge off contractions.

Massage exercises with a partner

With a partner, your husband or whomever you find suitable, practise the following three massages. The best position to be massaged in is the resting position (page 35) sitting on a chair reversed around and leaning on its back rest. In it, your lower back and thighs are well placed to be massaged by your partner.

1 Your partner should first of all massage your back, especially the lower back area. He or she should firmly knead and use friction (i.e. pressure using fingers and thumbs) around the base of your spinal column. For example, making small arches with the heel of the hand on the sacrum is extremely helpful. It's pure common sense. Find the parts that are sensitive, and firmly but gently massage these painful parts until the ache subsides. This may be done wherever you tend to tense up, neck, shoulders, and so on. Your partner should become familiar with your tense spots during pregnancy and so be able to recognize them when you are in labour and know what to do.

2 The second part to be massaged is your thighs. Your partner should place both hands around the top of your thighs and pull lightly from your upper thighs along your thigh to your knee. Then letting go, he should draw his or her hands back along your thigh to your upper thigh with no pressure at all; then again along your thigh from upper thigh to knee.

3 The third massage is that of your lower belly. Your partner should lightly put his or her finger tips on your abdomen, curve the fingers around in an arch from one side of your pubic bone to the other without completing the circle.

The first two massages should take about five to ten minutes each and the last one two or three minutes.

You will find in massaging your own body well that it is possible to massage painful spots away, that it stimulates and soothes your tissues and is pleasurable. When you are massaged by another person the same things happen and if your partner is good at it, all these effects may be enhanced. Everyone enjoys having her or his back scratched and to be massaged at the right time by the right person constitutes one of the supreme pleasures.

To be touched or massaged by another is more than physical stimulation or soothing. It may also be a communication of affection, assurance, comfort, acceptance or togetherness, and the pleasures from these may be mentally and emotionally relaxing, which is invaluable. There is possibly no better time, for some women, to receive affection and assurance than when in labour.

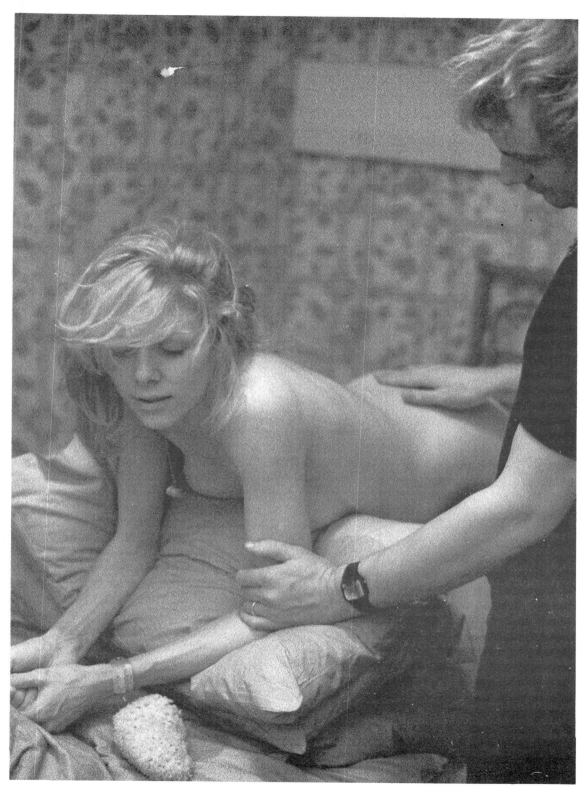

Massaging the lower back during a
contraction

10 Suggested programme during pregnancy

Throughout the book there are about thirty suggested movements, positions, and exercises to be practised during pregnancy. They may be divided into four groups.

1 Exploration of your body

Two simple pelvic exercises, (1) establishes the sense of your pelvis as a funnel (page 25), and (2) establishes the sense of your pelvic muscles (page 26). *See also* self-examination and massage (page 86).

These can be done daily after bath, shower or washing yourself, and should not take more than ten to fifteen minutes.

2 Pelvic control

Pelvic uptilt (page 54). Alternate closing and resting of your pelvic floor (page 56).

These exercises are designed to make you aware of your pelvic floor muscles and to make them more stable in pregnancy and more stretchable in childbirth. They can be done anytime and in various positions and should not take more than five minutes.

3 Relaxation

There are about twenty relaxing positional exercises.

Resting positions (page 33).

Squatting (page 70)

Sitting on your heels with knees apart (page 40)

And variation going forward

All-fours (page 42)

Knee-chest (page 42)

Tailor position (page 43)

Tailor position on a wall (page 44)

Legs apart on a wall (page 45)

Squatting on a wall (page 46)

Sitting between your feet with knees apart (page 47)

Twisting (page 50)

Sitting with your legs apart (page 51)

Tailor position, lying on your back (page 52)

And variation

Bending forward from standing position (page 53)

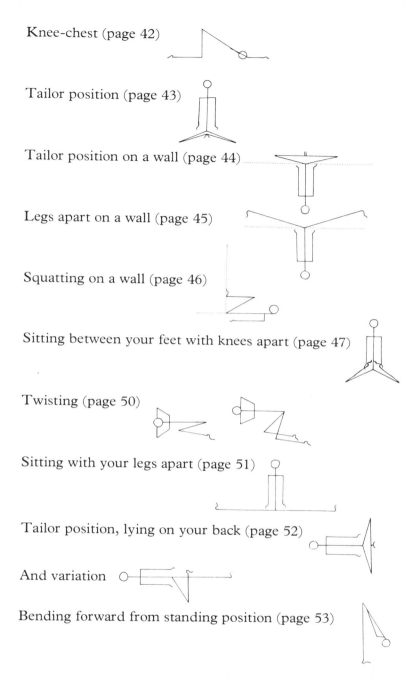

To begin with you need at least thirty minutes each day gradually to make yourself familiar with these exercises. Within two months you should be able to maintain each position with ease for five minutes.

4 Breathing
Your breathing will improve with practise. Set aside a few

minutes each day and follow the exercises recommended in Chapter 7.

You will find that over several weeks or months you will have cultivated a deeply effective way to centre, calm and relax yourself.

Practise deep breathing while resting, squatting, kneeling or stretching. The earlier in pregnancy you begin the exercises the better.

Minimum adequate relaxation programme
Thirty minutes each day. Start with two and a half minutes in a resting position, then five minutes squatting, five minutes kneeling and bending forwards, five minutes on all-fours, plus five minutes for *one* of the other relaxing positional exercises, varying the choice each session. End with five minutes squatting and two and a half minutes in the resting position.

Maximum relaxation programme, given time and inclination
Eighty-five minutes each day. Start with two and a half minutes resting, then five minutes squatting, five minutes on *all* the other relaxing positions and end with five minutes squatting and two and a half minutes resting.

Last six weeks of pregnancy
Time should be found at least once a week.
1 To practise deep breathing while imagining uterine contractions during the different stages of labour (Chapter 7).
2 To have your thighs and lower back massaged (page 88).
For both you will need the help of another person. Fifteen minutes should be set aside for the breathing practice and fifteen minutes for the massage.
3 All six positions recommended for labour (pages 66–9).

Doing exercises in company may be more inspiring than doing them alone
At times it may be fun to have your husband, friend or friends willing to work with you in cultivating many of these exercises. You may have a friend who is also pregnant or who wishes someday to become pregnant and sees the good sense in overcoming stiff pelvic joints and muscles.

If you are assisting your partner to further his or her range of movement, never push or use force: with your hands or legs just use your weight gradually, smoothly, and gently in the appropriate place. Never use jerky movements, but lever or lean your weight slowly. The person being assisted should always be the guide to how much weight is needed. In the photographs that follow, ways of promoting movement in particular positions are shown. They should be attempted only when both partners are familiar with the exercises and have cultivated them to a reasonable degree on their own.

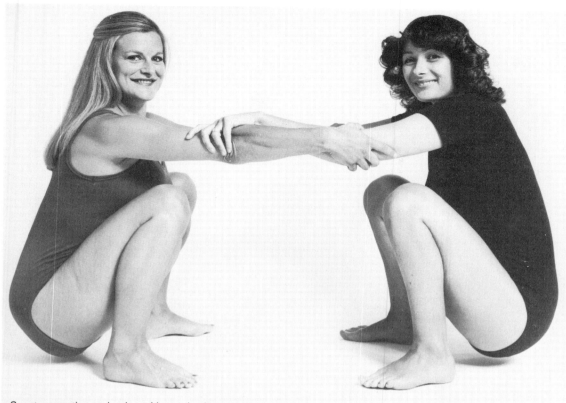

Squat supporting each other with your heels on the floor

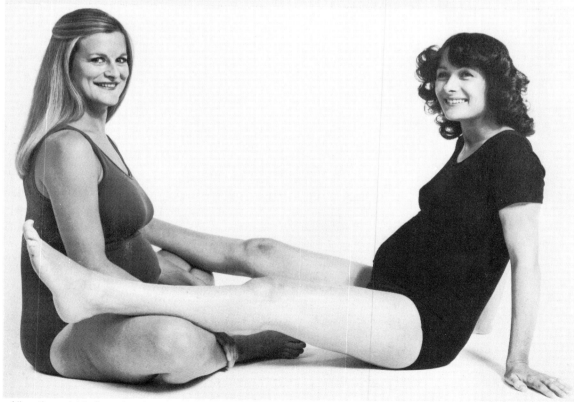

Allow the weight of your legs to promote your partner's movement

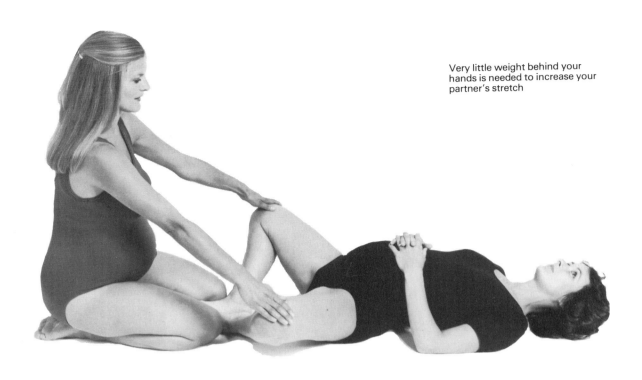

Very little weight behind your
hands is needed to increase your
partner's stretch

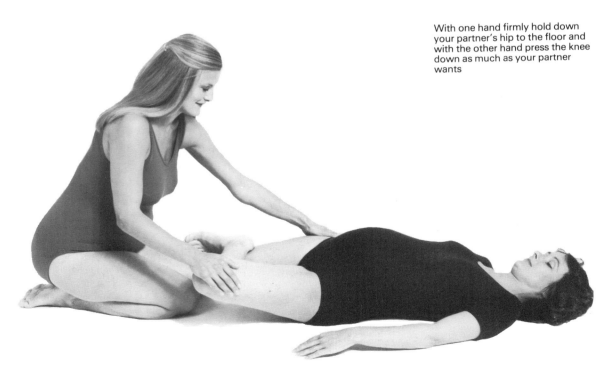

With one hand firmly hold down
your partner's hip to the floor and
with the other hand press the knee
down as much as your partner
wants

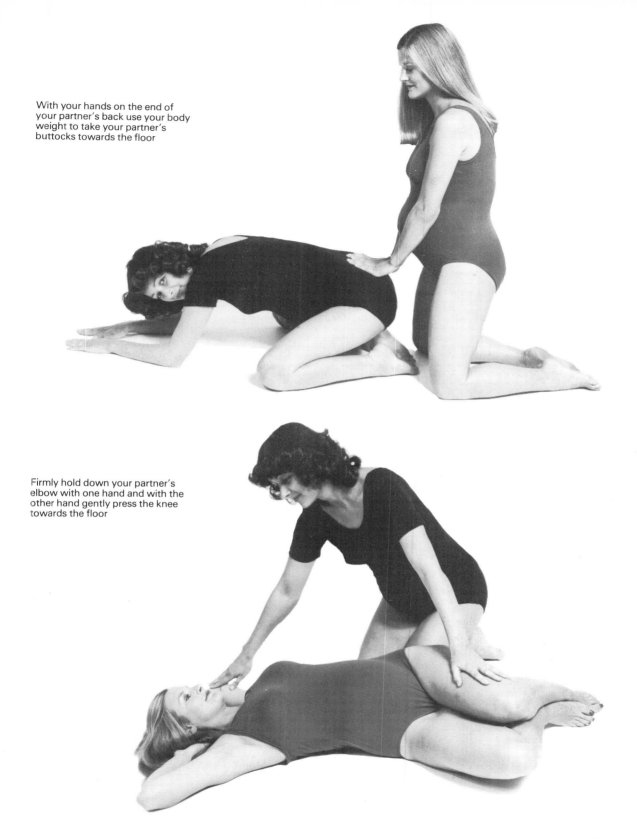

With your hands on the end of
your partner's back use your body
weight to take your partner's
buttocks towards the floor

Firmly hold down your partner's
elbow with one hand and with the
other hand gently press the knee
towards the floor

11 Labour and birth

With the increased understanding and control of your body that have been achieved by the exercises carried out during pregnancy, you approach labour with confidence. The whole point of these months of preparation is the birth of your child: you have done your best to be at your best.

This chapter now takes you through the main processes of labour and delivery. It starts with an explanation of what happens during contractions, both the workings of your unseen muscles and the feelings of pain and pleasure you may experience from them. The causes and significance of pain in labour are then considered. The rest of the chapter is taken up with describing what is happening to you at the various stages of labour, following the progress of your child in the last hours before being born, and suggesting ways, largely by the choice of bodily positions and breathing movements, that will help both you and your child.

Throughout labour the main active forces involved are the contractions and retractions of muscular walls of your uterus. Other active forces are those of gravity and of increased intra-abdominal pressure from your breathing movements and the contractions of your abdominal muscles. These active forces are accompanied by the stretching and opening of your cervix, vagina, and pelvic floor. Obviously their passive yielding is as essential in allowing your child to be born as the contracting and retracting of the walls of the uterus.

Contractions and retractions explained

A contraction occurs when nerve impulses initiate a shortening or drawing together of the muscle fibres. When this happens you experience a tightening of your uterus. Throughout the greater part of pregnancy you will already have felt intermittent contractions passing over the body of your uterus from time to time. The contractions during labour are an exaggeration of these, but with the difference that the uterine muscle retracts as well as contracts. The result is that a certain amount of the shortening produced by each contraction is retained: the muscle fibres become shorter with each contraction and never stretch back quite to their original length. There is thus during labour a progressive shrinking in the capacity of the body of your uterus. This is one of the principal factors in the opening of the cervix and the expelling of the child.

If you sense a contraction as only a tightening or closing action then you sense only half the action. Muscles, you will recall, work in opposing teams, so contractions involve the active closing of the upper part of your uterus and simultaneously a passive opening of the neck of your uterus.

How does a uterine contraction transmit its force?

As long as your cervix is undilated or closed, the force of a uterine contraction is applied equally in all directions (see diagram 1). If this continued there would be no progress in the birth of your child. However, your cervix softens and becomes an area of lessened resistance and thereafter the pressure of the foetal head and of the fluid in the uterus acts downwards on it (see diagrams 2 and 3).

After the rupture of the membranes surrounding your baby, much of the fluid may be held back if your child's head fits tightly into the lower part of your uterus and the uterine force will continue to be transmitted as a general fluid pressure. But if much of the fluid was drained, some of the force may then be directed downwards through the axis of your child.

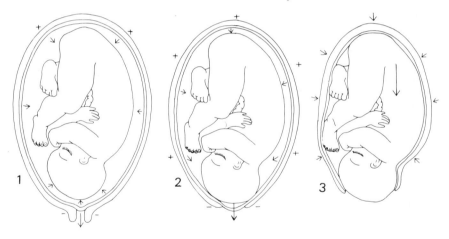

1   When the cervix is undilated, the force of a uterine contraction is applied equally in all directions

2   The cervix begins to open and the force of a uterine contraction acts downwards

3   The cervix is fully opened and the pressure of the fluid in the contracting uterus acts downward on the child

What happens during a contraction?

Most uterine contractions flow like waves through the whole of your uterus, beginning at the top and spreading downwards, getting stronger, reaching a peak, and then fading away. The beginning and end of contractions are not experienced, although by placing your hands on your abdomen you can feel a tightening or hardening. After one contraction has ceased there is an interval, followed by another contraction. As labour advances contractions become longer, stronger, and more frequent and the intervals between them shorter.

That the contractions are intermittent is of enormous value. In the intervals the pressure on your child and on your abdominal organs is relieved and the placental blood flow, which is slowed down at the peak of contraction, is restored.

1 In the standing position, the forward movement of the uterus as it contracts is not resisted by gravity

2 In the reclining position, the uterus must contract against gravity to elongate and move itself forward. This wastes much-needed energy

3 In the inclining position, the uterus is lined up without the need to move forwards during a contraction

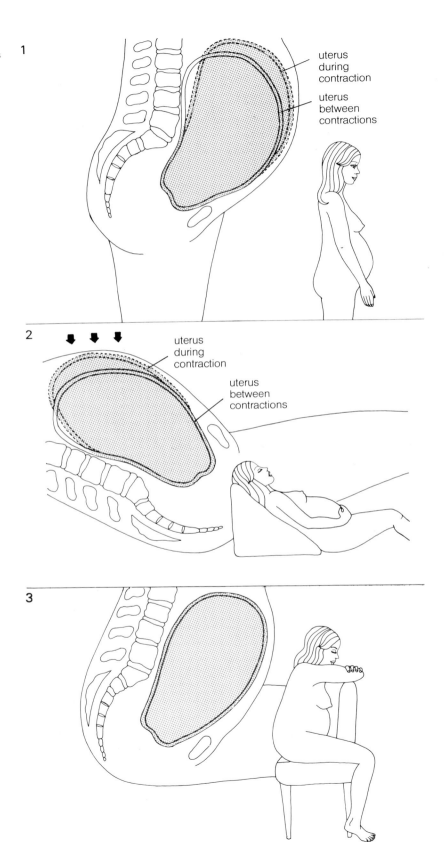

1

uterus during contraction

uterus between contractions

2

uterus during contraction

uterus between contractions

3

During a uterine contraction.
1 Your blood pressure is raised.
2 Your pulse rate is quickened.
3 Breathing is slowed at the height of a contraction.
4 Intra-uterine pressure is raised.
5 Your child's heartbeat reacts.
6 Your uterus narrows, elongates and rears itself slightly forward so that its long axis is brought to lie in the axis of your pelvic inlet (see diagram on the opposite page).

If you are lying down or leaning backwards, extra effort is demanded from your uterus to align itself against the force of gravity in every contraction. This extra effort over many hours may prove exhausting.

If you are upright and leaning forward during a contraction, less effort is needed. A sitting inclining position is best to aid the action of your uterus in every contraction. Your child takes the line of least resistance, and strenuous rearing forward of your uterus is unnecessary.

The contractions and retractions of your uterus are the cause of the intense feelings felt during labour: no uterine contraction, no intense feelings, either of pleasure or pain. Sometimes women do have constant dull backache or abdominal discomfort throughout labour, but these intensify only during contractions.

How these feelings arise

There are receptors in all the visceral muscles in your body and in your joints, tendons, and skeletal muscles, and they record stretching and contraction. The intense feelings during uterine contractions arise principally from the visceral muscle of your uterus and, at certain points in labour, from the joints and skeletal muscles of your pelvis. If skeletal or visceral muscle contracts and stretches only to a certain point, the feelings are pleasurable. Beyond that point, contracting and stretching of the muscles will cause pain.

In everyday life external sensations (such as sight, sound, smell, taste or feeling heat or cold) are predominant. But during labour internal sensations are in the foreground. Because this is unusual it can be frightening at first. Some of the characteristic sensations accompanying uterine contractions are the sense of pressure, sense of something to be expelled, sense of advance, sense of impending defecation, feelings of bearing down, and the sense of stretching or opening.

These sensations vary from woman to woman and this fact accounts for the widely different reaction to labour. Some women say it was the worst experience they ever had; others say it was mainly painful; others say mainly pleasurable, and others say it had its painful and pleasurable, if not ecstatic, moments. Pleasure and pain are clearly private subjective experiences and your experience may not be quite like anyone else's. For sure, we all feel pleasure and pain differently and there is no doubt that certain women are better able to handle intense sensations than others.

In a healthy undrugged woman intense feelings are inevitable in labour; how could it be otherwise in such a dynamic act as childbirth? But it seems strange that the intense sensations should so often be painful. Other comparable physiological functions are in health not only painless but pleasurable.

Your uterus is an organ, designed first to retain and then to expel its contents, just as are your lungs, bowel, bladder, and other hollow organs. In micturition and defecation there is at least the pleasure of relief of pressure, if not something much more positive. When the call to evacuate is satisfied there may be a feeling similar to elation. Animals seem to have pleasure in these functions, including labour. Cats, for example, often purr when their kittens are being born.

Some women also give birth without any, or at most inconsiderable, pain. Labour is gone through accompanied by a sense of powerful pressure, a sense of stretching and opening fully, the desire to strain as at stool and so on, but without any sensations that could be considered as pain. But for a great many women pain in labour is real enough and the suffering involved should not be underestimated. This you may willingly bear as something not nearly so important as the birth of your child. Whatever pains and discomforts you may have experienced, if you and your child are uninjured and healthy at the end of childbirth it has been a total success. This pleasure in the end outweighs all the pain suffered to reach it.

Organic and functional pain
You must distinguish between two kinds of pain, organic pain and functional pain. Organic pain comes from some kind of damage to tissues or from disease, whereas functional pain arises without evidence of any injury or disease. Most of the pain experienced in labour is functional; it inflicts no injury and a sense of ease, even of satisfaction, may be felt when it has passed. There is one exception, that is in the final expulsive stage when the delicate tissues of the perineum may tear slightly, causing damage and therefore organic pain.

Pain as a message
Pain always has a reason behind it. It is a message that something is amiss. For example, if you tread on a sharp point with your bare foot the pain from it is a warning signal and you quickly withdraw your foot. So, although we all dislike and avoid pain, we would not be better off without the ability to experience it. It is not always an evil thing that must be driven away by drugs. More often than not we are in pain because we need to be in pain. People who have no pain receptors in their skin, and there are such people, cannot protect themselves from

danger. They severely burn themselves, gravely injure their heads and limbs, because they do not get the early warning signal of pain.

Pain is also felt when physiological needs are not met and is a warning signal that these needs, such as emptying the bladder or bowels, must be satisfied. There is no physiological function in health that gives rise to pain unless the need to perform is frustrated. This is true in childbirth. The pain in labour is a warning signal that parts of the body are somehow resisting the process of childbirth.

During pregnancy the muscle fibres of the cervix and the muscles surrounding the vagina remain contracted, firmly closed, retaining the contents of the uterus. As labour begins, the muscles of the cervical and vaginal outlets are relaxed, and the natural course of events is for pressure within the uterus to build up causing dilation of first the cervix and then the vagina and its surrounding muscles. But if the cervix and birth canal do not give sufficiently, the pressure within the uterus may build up to acute pain at the height of a contraction. This is the pain of excessive intra-uterine pressure and results in fatigue.

Pain may also arise at the height of the dilation of the cervix in its first stage of labour, and at the height of the dilation of the perineum in the second stage of labour because of resistance within the muscles themselves to the full stretching that allows the child to pass through to be born.

'Rain, after all, is only rain; it is not bad weather. So also pain is only pain; unless we resist it, when it becomes torment.'

I Ching

Labour and delivery

With a clearer understanding of what happens during contractions and of the intense sensations associated with labour it is now possible to trace the various stages of labour and delivery. No birth is ever quite like another, as any woman who has had several children knows. But the main process of birth is fairly predictable and a mother who has prepared herself during pregnancy to be at her best for childbirth can more readily cope with any minor variations. The course of exercises you have been following will have helped you through pregnancy itself, but it is in childbirth that they really pay off.

Labour goes through a variety of stages.

1 First-stage labour (dilation of the cervix) and transition stage (dilation of the cervix completed).

2 Second-stage labour (expulsion of the child begins) and perineum stage (delivery of the child).

3 Third-stage labour (delivery of the placenta).

The following guide outlines what is happening inside your body, what is happening to your child, and what you can do to help in its delivery through use of the techniques you have mastered during pregnancy.

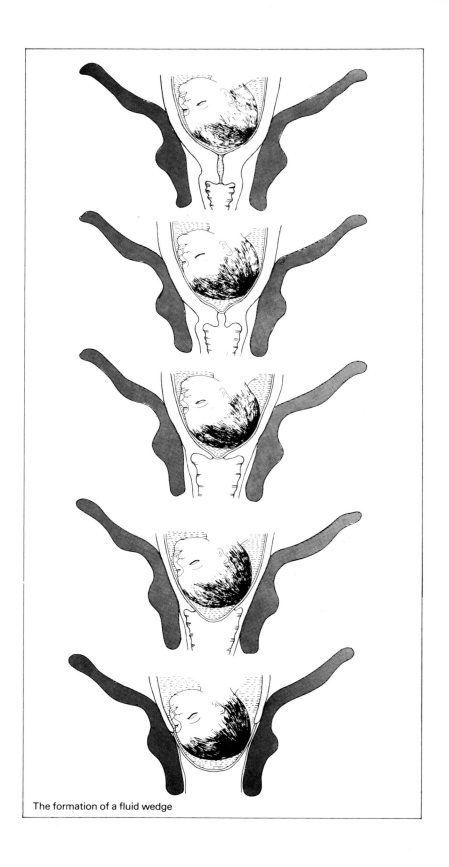

The formation of a fluid wedge

The first stage

What is happening to you?

Delivery of your child cannot begin until two things have happened. First, the lower part of the body of your uterus, known as the lower uterine segment, has to become stretched and thinned and secondly, the neck of the uterus, the cervix, has to dilate and open.

The explanation of this is that a hollow organ like your uterus can expel its contents only if one part of it is weaker than the rest. Otherwise contractions would merely raise pressure in the organ without leading to any expulsion of its contents. In the uterus the weak spot is the cervix.

During pregnancy the body of your uterus is in a state of relaxation, stretching and opening (except for those slight intermittent contractions) and your cervix is in a state of contraction. During labour the reverse happens, the body of your uterus contracts and your cervix relaxes, stretches, and opens.

The weakness of the lower uterine segment largely results from its design. The muscle fibres are mostly longitudinal without many transverse fibres to give strength and cohesion. The thinning begins towards the end of pregnancy and the segment is further progressively stretched when labour starts.

The show

When the lower uterine segment is stretched and its surface area enlarged, the attached membranes are separated. This is the reason for the mucous discharge in labour known as the 'show'.

The formation of a fluid wedge (the bag of waters)

As soon as the opening between the body of the uterus and cervix begins to expand, the membranes and their fluid contents bulge into the opening. Each successive contraction makes them protrude more into the proper part of your cervix and in this way they act as a fluid wedge increasing the diameter of your cervix.

Your entire cervix is expanded and stretched into a funnel before its opening into your vagina begins to enlarge. The elasticity of the membranes often keeps them intact until your cervix is fully dilated, but the rupture of the membranes may occur before that, causing the escape of the fluid wedge (forewaters).

What your sensations may be

Contractions come like waves and the early contractions may sometimes be more difficult than those later ones, not because they are stronger, but because you have not had time to adjust to them, especially if it is your first birth. The pain of the early first stage is most often described as rather like a period pain, a sort of tightening, slightly aching feeling in the lower abdominal area and across the tops of the thighs.

Between the time when the cervix is two-thirds dilated and the end of the first stage, contractions become faster and stronger. Sensations may be overpowering but can be at the same time pleasurable. Your body takes over. They are certainly often quite bearable. The stronger they get the more frequently they come with acute abdominal tightening and pressure.

You may feel the sensations in the body of your uterus or you may experience a concentration of feeling over the neck (cervix) of the uterus. Sometimes there are aches and pain in the small of your back. The contraction of the uterus itself may cause pain, especially if it is against strong resistance. Pain may also be caused by the thinning out, stretching and opening of your cervix that occurs at the height of contractions. The pain from this may spread to your groins and inner thighs and sometimes muscle cramps occur in them. You may experience a pulling or tightening feeling going from your pubic joint in front to your sacrum at the back. It is ring-like and pulls together tighter and tighter at the peak of contraction.

Earlier in the chapter it was emphasized that pain during labour is a message that parts of your body are resisting. The message should be heeded. Pains in the first stage of dilation may be signals to make sure that your body's skeletal system is relaxed in an appropriate resting position. They may be demanding a change of position to one more suitable. Or they may be messages to control your breathing movements.

Gradually the nature of contractions changes, perhaps becoming more irregular. As your cervix fully dilates and your uterus prepares to expel its contents, the desire to bear down begins to be experienced. This phase is often accompanied by backache, or a feeling of anal pressure, and for some may be the most painful time. The message of pain in the transitional stage may be that you should slow down and allow full dilation of your cervix before going on with your bearing down impulses.

What you can do to help: (1) Positions
During the early part of the first stage there is little active work you can do to aid the dilation of your cervix. Your uterus, like your heart or liver, operates independently of thought and will, and continues to work without your intervention. Generally, you should remain up and about, waiting for the contractions to increase in frequency.

Allow your body to go with the involuntary process going on inside you. Focus your attention on the sensations coming from your uterus and the surrounding skeletal muscles. There is nothing to escape from, nothing to avoid, nothing to oppose, and nothing you cannot face or cope with or go through. Each contraction brings you closer to the goal of birth.

Once labour is fully established and your cervix begins to open or dilate, uterine contractions last about a minute, with about five minutes or so of inactivity in between. During contractions you can use the resting position or any other position you find suitable. Resting is of the greatest aid during this time and if you are good at it you may avoid unnecessary discomfort. Immediately there is a sign of a contraction, assume a comfortable resting position in which your skeletal muscles are inactive and relaxed. Besides the contraction of your uterus, you do not need contraction elsewhere in your body. Unnecessary muscle contractions make labour more difficult, fatiguing, and longer. Check that you are not tightening or contracting any muscles unduly.

During the first stage it is not advisable to lie flat on your back for too long. Upright positions assist the dilation of your cervix and improve the flow of blood through your uterus, providing more oxygen for your child. These are the main advantages in remaining upright and about. Left to your own freedom, you will probably adopt many different positions in this first stage. If back pain or any other discomfort persists during contractions, several positons may be tried to discover the best, by trial and error. One of them may relieve discomfort or pressure on your back.

If you find it comforting to be touched and massaged by someone who cares for you, don't hesitate to ask to be massaged at any time during labour. This is often very relaxing to many women and to some it is vital. They feel in contact, encouraged and not alone. Others don't want to be massaged or touched in any way during labour and feel in contact through other ways. Moving your body rhythmically, rotating or rocking your hips, may be very helpful. In many cultures women are taught a dance to be done during pregnancy and birth. This can be a very enjoyable way to release tension and dissipate pain. You may also find it helpful to have a warm bath and to try some of these positions in the water. Immersion in warm water is particularly helpful if the dilation is slow or if the labour is difficult.

Transition Stage: the last part of the first stage, known as the transition stage, is often the most intense and difficult part of the labour. Your cervix is completing its dilation and the body of your uterus is preparing to expel your child. Uterine contractions last about one and a half minutes with short intervals between them of half a minute to one minute. The transition stage can last only a few minutes or as much as two or three hours.

While the dilation of your cervix is completing, you may begin to feel the urge to push or bear down. This may be accompanied by intense feelings of anal pressure as your child's head presses down against the back of the birth canal. Adopt any position that helps you. If you need to speed up the process during contractions, squatting or kneeling or standing are appropriate, but it is more likely that you will need to slow down. This is because of the risk of beginning the expulsive second stage too early, before your cervix is quite fully opened. What might then happen is that the front lip of your cervix (anterior lip) could get caught up and block the exit. To slow down, or to have more control, the all-fours position is most useful. Many women instinctively use this position during transition. To help control the urge to push in the case of an anterior lip use the knee chest position for three or four contractions. This will slow down the activity of your uterus and abdominal muscles and will lessen the force of gravity until your cervix is fully dilated and the second stage may safely begin.

What you can do to help: (2) Breathing

During the greater part of all stages of labour the most useful skill to use is your ability to be aware of your breathing without interfering with it. But if you begin to feel overwhelmed by the intensity of the contractions, use your will to breathe deeply by concentrating on the exhalation and allowing the inhalation to come of its own accord.

Transition stage: you will probably find that as you approach the end of the first stage you will be breathing more heavily and making more noise. Slowing down, if needed at this stage, can be done by breathing very deeply and slowly and concentrating on the exhalation. However, some women find more shallow breathing helpful at this stage. Whether the breathing is deep or shallow, quiet or noisy, concentrating on the exhalation will help to release tension.

What is happening to your child?

Ninety-five per cent of babies are born with their heads first. Your child's head is relatively large and, as we have seen, it has to pass through the bony structure of the pelvic canal. The principal difficulties in doing this are the curve of the pelvic canal and the spirals and twists in it.

In the last weeks of pregnancy the lower uterine segment stretches to accept your child's head as it descends into your pelvis. This is known as engagement, your child's head tends to be flexed on its neck, and the vertex, which is the crown of its head, becomes the part lowest in the birth canal. (Occiput refers to the back part and sinciput to the front part of the head.)

Before labour begins the crown of your child's head fits into the inlet of your pelvic canal. Its head lies in the side-to-side diameter of your pelvis, that is, it is facing towards the left or right of your pelvis. During the first stage of labour, through contraction and retraction of your uterus, your child descends slightly, with further flexion of its head.

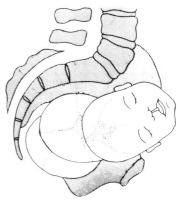

The flexed head is engaged facing towards the left or right side of the pelvis

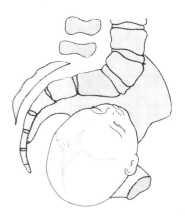

As the head descends, it rotates

The second stage

What is happening to you

The second stage begins when the cervix has been completely dilated, and the child's head moves into the birth canal. This stage ends with the perineum stage when your child is born.

The contractions of the uterus continue and their expulsive action is helped by contractions of your abdominal muscles and the muscles of your diaphragm. Both of these increase intra-abdominal pressure. To a much lesser degree the force of gravity also aids your uterus.

To be born, your child will have to pass through your pelvic floor. From the point of view of its action in childbirth your pelvic floor can be regarded as being made up of two parts that act like shutters. The front pubic part lies within your subpubic arch; the back sacral part is attached to your buttock bones and your coccyx and sacrum. When the two shutters open in childbirth, the pubic part is pulled inwards and the sacral part is pushed outwards.

The pubic part has comparatively few voluntary muscles connecting it to your pubic bones, whereas the sacral part has almost ninety per cent of all the pelvic floor muscles connected to it. So in childbirth it is the back sacral part that has to give, to stretch back, to make room for your child's head and body, and not the front pubic part. To be free to move backwards when pressure is applied your sacrum, and the sacral area of your pelvic floor, must be in a passive state of stretching.

The position of your body at this stage is all important. If you are lying on your back, your sacrum is not free to move backwards and the back sacral part of your pelvic floor is not in a passive stretching state. This forces your child's head to press forwards towards the bony subpubic arch instead of backwards towards your sacrum and coccyx, which are mobile and extendable.

But if you are squatting or kneeling or inclining, the position of your pelvis is altered. Your pubic bones are lifted up in front and your sacrum and coccyx extended back. Your back sacral area is in a passive stretching state and if your child's head presses against this, it passively stretches further backwards, making room and allowing as much give as possible.

What your sensations may be

There are great variations in the length of the first and second stages in different women and also the amount of pressure and suffering accompanying them. A short first stage tends to be followed by a short second stage, whereas a long first stage may be succeeded by a short, medium, or long second stage, ranging between two or three minutes and as many hours.

The second stage is commonly more endurable than the first and is indeed often enjoyable. The pleasure it brings is similar

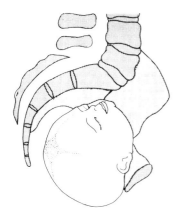

The head rotates until it faces the sacrum

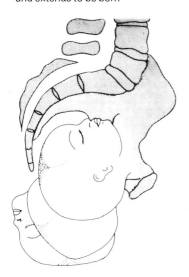

Finally, the head descends and extends to be born

107

to the simple enjoyment in defecation. The urge to push may be irresistible and the muscular effort is often pleasant. Pressure at this stage builds up enormously and any resistance at the outlet to the expulsive effort causes discomfort and pain. However, the intense and extraordinary sensations of the descent of your child's head can not only be painless but positively satisfying.

The perineum stage : for some women the crowning of the infant's head is one of the most painful moments of childbirth; they do not find these last few moments pleasant. The feeling of being about to pop or tear predominates. In this stage you will begin to feel yourself gradually opening up. This often comes with a tingling sensation as your perineum bulges and may be very acute. Some women dislike this feeling intensely; others like it.

If you push down hard insensitively and do not wait for the gradual dilation of your perineum, you are likely to experience pain and perhaps slight tearing of your perineum. The crowning of your child's head, its birth, and the birth of the rest of its body should all take place slowly and gradually. The pain of stretching the perineum is rather like that you feel when you pull at the corners of your mouth with your fingers.

The message of pain in the first part of the second stage may stimulate you to assist in pushing out your child by regular pressure of your abdominal muscles. Pains in the perineum stage may be urging you to slow down to prevent too fast a birth and the tearing of your tissues.

A painless and pleasurable labour resembles the average labour in every respect, except in the absence of pain during uterine contractions. The signs are just the same – 'show', flow of waters, dilation of vagina and perineum, and the various durations of the individual stages of labour.

What you can do to help: (1) Positions
You neither need to relax nor can you do so by resting during the expulsive uterine contractions of the second stage. They last about half a minute to a minute with about two to three minutes of rest in between. The skeletal muscles that assist your baby through the birth canal come into play strongly. This involves total physical exertion, deep breaths are drawn and the effort is just as great as any other strong physical activity.

This is the time when you can most actively participate in labour, and you should choose the position in which you can work best, changing at any time if you wish. In squatting and kneeling, your uterine contractions, plus the contractions of your abdominal muscles and diaphragm, will in most instances push your child's head down on to your perineum without very great physical effort on your part. If you are reclining, you may tire more rapidly because the task of your uterus is made more difficult.

There are various ways in which you can be supported squatting in the second stage. You could squat on your toes and hold on to a support in front of you. You could be supported by two people kneeling on either side of you, using their knees beneath your buttocks for support. A partner could sit behind you on a chair with you squatting between his knees. Alternatively, your partner could stand and you could be supported from behind in a 'standing squat'. In this case your partner should take care not to stoop but should carry your weight against his pelvis, bending his knees, tightening his buttocks and leaning back a little. You could also face him and place your arms around his neck in which case the midwife would receive the baby from behind.

It is important to try out all these positions when you are pregnant in order to be able to use them without difficulty in labour.

Any kneeling position is suitable for birth and is particularly useful in the case of a very fast second stage when the 'all-fours' position will give you a sense of control and help to slow down the contractions a little.

Rest and relax completely between contractions in the kneeling position, supporting your head and arms on a chair or bed. This is the most effective way of recuperating muscle power.

The more you can assist your uterus, from above by the action of your abdominal wall and diaphragm and from below by adopting a position that allows your pelvic muscles to stretch passively and open your pelvic floor, the easier your child will be born. Squatting and kneeling encourage both. They reduce the intra-abdominal space above and relax and open your pelvic floor muscles as well as your buttock and sacral muscles.

The perineum or delivery stage
Towards the end of the second stage your baby's head crowns and descends on to the perineum, which dilates and stretches to allow the head to pass through. This can happen quite effortlessly, but sometimes considerable difficulty is experienced accompanied by a sensation of stretching and bursting.

It is helpful to restrain all voluntary effort and to allow the vulnerable perineal tissues to gradually stretch open, using a kneeling or supported squatting position – in which this part of your body is most relaxed and gravity is helping to ease your baby out.

In between the final contractions, after your baby's head has crowned, you should try to be as relaxed as possible in your chosen position. The last contraction or two give birth to your child's head. This is a crucial stage. Make sure that you are not unwittingly willing your pelvic floor to close by tightening your anus and vagina.

How you can help: (2) Breathing
Some women enjoy working with the urges to bear down and

others prefer simply to let go and let their uterus do all the work. Either way, when you feel a contraction coming on, take a deep breath and then bear down or let go as you breathe out. Never hold your breath as this slows down your circulation, reducing the blood supply to your uterus and thus to your baby. Many women feel a need to cry out or scream as they bear down, and say that this helps them to relax and release the baby.

What is happening to your child?
After the full dilation of the cervix, the contractions (aided by contractions of your abdominal muscles and diaphragm) force your child's head to descend to the level of the middle of your pelvic canal. At this point rotation begins as its head meets the grooved gutter of your pelvic floor.

Descent continues and further flexion of the head occurs and the back of the head rotates to the front through about ninety degrees. After the rotation, which takes time, the back of the head lies in the front behind your pubic joint.

The head emerges

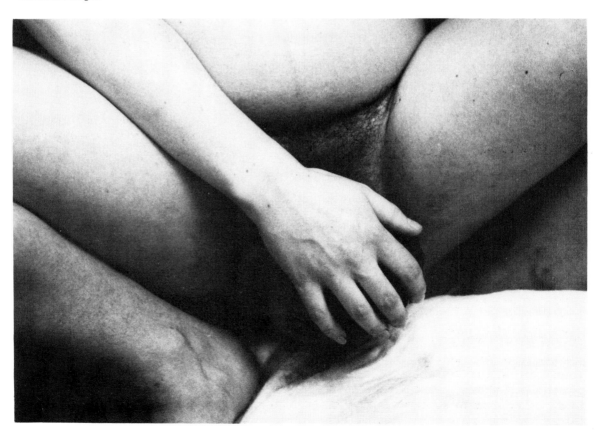

More propulsive contractions, aided by increased intra-abdominal pressure, force your child's head further down towards your vulva. (Although the rotation is usually complete before the back of its head reaches your vulva, it may not be completed until the actual expulsion, with your child's head still turning as it is born.) Then the crown of its head appears, stretching your vaginal opening. With further contractions its head emerges and its face sweeps under your perineum.

At this point the shoulders of your child have now reached your pelvic floor and they are rotated (as its head has just done) to lie in the front-to-back diameter of your pelvic canal's outlet. The head therefore now rotates in the opposite direction and returns to the position it held at the onset of labour.

The birth of the shoulders takes place by bending to the sides. First they bend backwards, to free the front shoulder from behind your pubic joint, and then forwards to free the back shoulder. With both shoulders born the rest of your child's body is rapidly expelled and born.

In passing through your pelvis your child's head has been subjected to considerable pressure from both the hard and soft passages. That the descent is done without damage to the head is made possible by the softness of the bones themselves and because the edges of the skull bones are membranous (i.e. made of soft tissue) and are separated from each other by very definite spaces so that they are able to overlap very slightly.

You will have made your child's descent easier if you have properly exercised your pelvic joints and their muscles during pregnancy, so allowing you to position your pelvis at its widest during labour. The fit between your child's head and your pelvis is so exact that the smallest increase in size of your pelvis during labour is significant.

The third stage

Immediately after giving birth, sit in an upright position, rather than lying back, as this will allow perfect first contact between you and your baby. When your child has begun to breathe, the placenta will no longer be needed and will separate from the wall of your uterus. Fifteen to thirty minutes after the birth there are usually more contractions, stimulated by the first sucking of your baby at the breast. These contractions will expel the placenta and membranes (afterbirth). There is very little for you to do other than to squat or stand, let go, and relax as the placenta comes out.

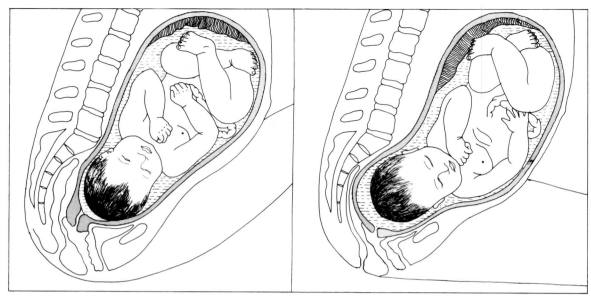

Late pregnancy The head has engaged in the pelvic inlet. The cervix is soft but has not thinned out

Early labour The head has moved more deeply into the pelvic canal. The cervix has thinned out but has not yet begun to dilate.

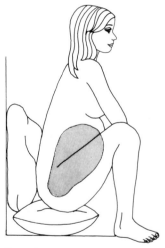

Squatting

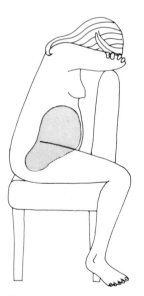

Resting on the back of a chair

Stages of labour

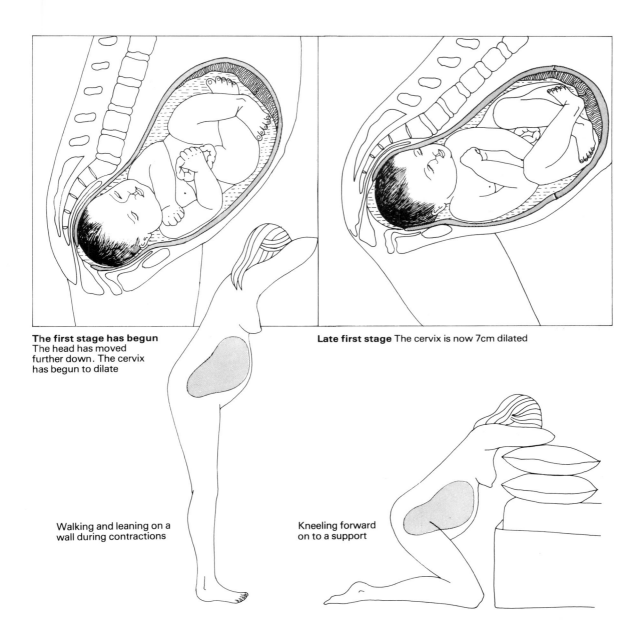

The first stage has begun
The head has moved
further down. The cervix
has begun to dilate

Late first stage The cervix is now 7cm dilated

Walking and leaning on a
wall during contractions

Kneeling forward
on to a support

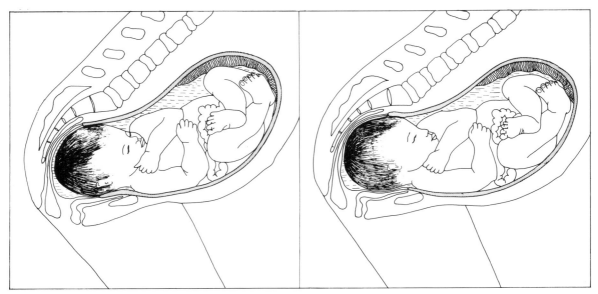

Transition The cervix is almost fully dilated and the head is beginning to rotate

Early second stage Dilation of the cervix is complete and the second stage is about to begin

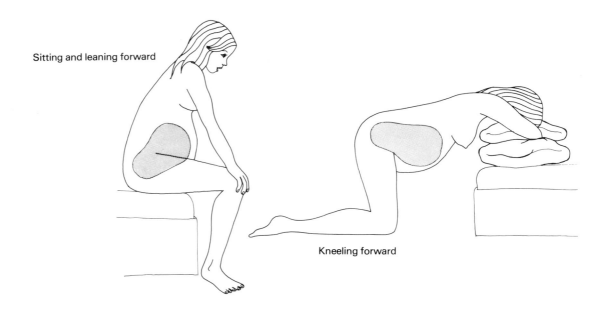

Sitting and leaning forward

Kneeling forward

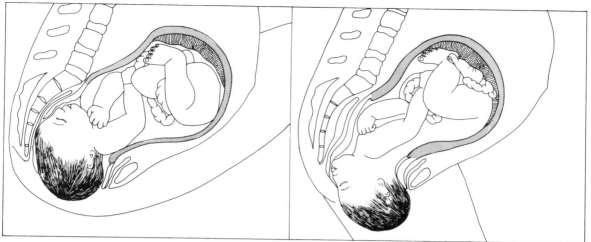

The head is crowning

Birth of the head

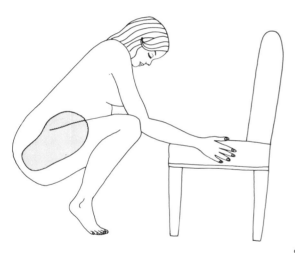

Squatting for bearing down,
holding on to a chair

Kneeling and leaning forward
on to a chair for bearing down

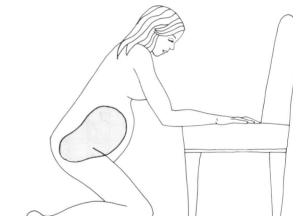

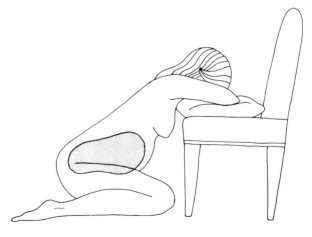

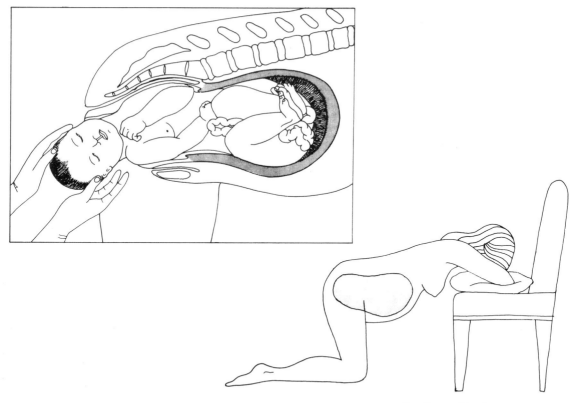

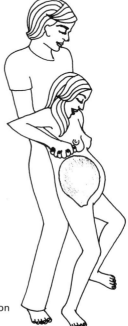

Kneeling position for delivery

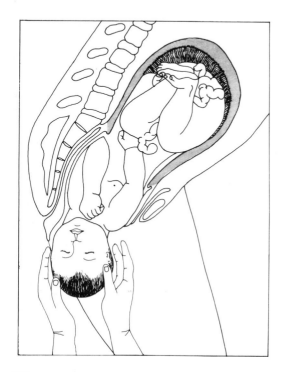

Supported standing position

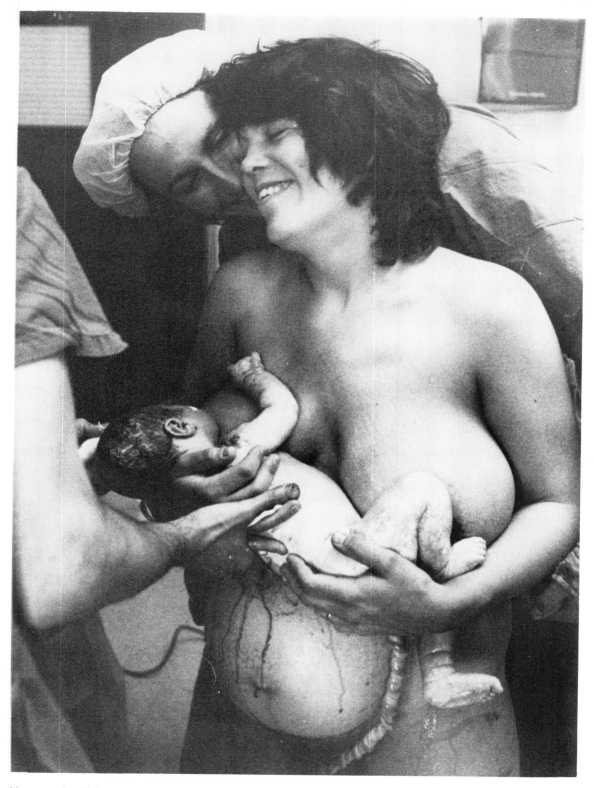

Moments after birth

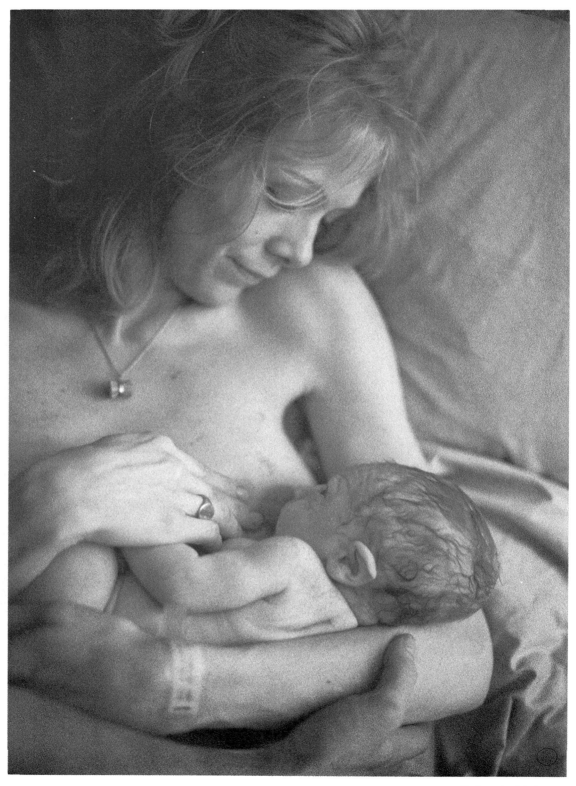

First contact between
mother and baby

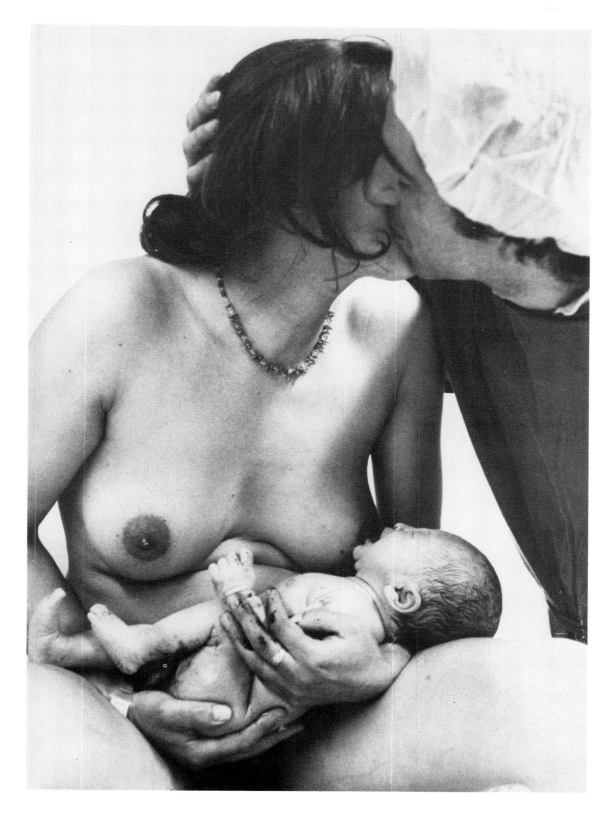

12 After the birth

The first hour

A moment or two after giving birth you will probably be holding your newborn baby in your arms and gazing for the first time into his or her eyes. This first contact between you happens, if circumstances allow, immediately after the birth before the completion of the third stage. This early period has been extensively researched in recent years, and it is now generally accepted that this is a vital time for 'bonding' to take place between you and your baby and the other members of the family. Many studies have shown that when this first contact is undisturbed the relationship between the mother and her child is much easier. Good bonding leads to good mothering and better contact between you and your baby. There is a natural symbiosis between you both. The presence of your baby releases your maternal instincts. The rush of emotion you feel as you gaze at your baby, the touch of his skin against yours, the sound of his cries, his first contact and suckling at your breast, all stimulate the contractions of the uterus. This causes the placenta to separate from the wall of the uterus and be delivered within the first half hour or so after the birth.

This process is helped if you are sitting really upright immediately after birth, rather than being propped up by pillows in a semi-reclining position, but you may need some support for your back. By sitting upright you can handle your baby easily. Skin to skin, eye to eye, mouth to nipple contact is perfect. This position is also safest and most favourable for the separation of the placenta and reduces the risk of excessive bleeding or haemorrage.

The newborn baby is acutely sensitive and alert in the first moments after birth. This is a very important time for your baby in which he or she will be making the transition from the womb to the outside world.

Used to being in water, your baby will be feeling the atmosphere on his skin, seeing light for the first time, smelling new smells and beginning to breathe. Your baby may appear slightly blue or grey in colour for a few moments after birth until he begins breathing. His head may be a little pointed in shape or 'moulded' after the journey through the pelvic canal. The skull bones overlap to facilitate this passage causing this moulding which will round out within a few hours of the birth. Your baby's body may also be covered in a white creamy substance known as vernix. This protects the baby from the change in temperature and is also a source of nourishment and is absorbed into the baby's body within a few hours.

Within minutes after birth the amniotic fluid in the baby's lungs is absorbed and air is inhaled and exhaled. While this is happening the placenta is still attached to the wall of your uterus and your baby is still receiving a good supply of blood from the umbilical cord. As soon as his breathing is properly established the cord will stop pulsating and the placenta, no longer needed, will begin to separate from the wall of the uterus. A good supply of oxygen is vital at this time. Nature has provided the baby with this double lifeline in order to help him make this transition safely. The cord normally stops pulsating within ten minutes after birth, and should not be clamped or cut until its function is completed.

During the first hour or two of his life your baby will be most alert but after this, in the days to come, he will probably be quite sleepy most of the time. Some families enjoy giving the newborn baby a bath in this first hour or two, and it can be a deeply enjoyable experience for all concerned and very relaxing for the baby. The water should be pleasantly warm and as deep as possible, so that the whole body of the baby is immersed. The purpose of this bath is for pleasure, rather than to clean the baby. It is not necessary to bathe the baby at all.

The baby can be bathed a few moments after birth, before the placenta is delivered, by placing the bath between the mother's legs on the floor, so that she can sit upright and, perhaps together with the father, bathe the baby. Or the baby can be bathed at any time that seems right.

Some mothers prefer to take the baby with them into a bath, and this is often a very pleasant way to include a toddler and introduce him or her to the new baby.

After breathing is well established, your baby gradually makes a transition from the placenta as its source of nourishment to its new lifeline – your breast. As well as the reflex to breathe, your baby has a powerful instinct to find the nipple, known as a 'rooting reflex'. By sitting upright and simply holding your baby in your arms he will feel your breast against his cheek and turn his head towards it to find the nipple and he will probably want to begin to suckle. Some babies take a while to actually start sucking whereas others take to the breast immediately. This first sucking within the first hour helps to facilitate successful breast-feeding, and also stimulates your body to release the hormones which contract the uterus and help to expel the placenta.

The days following the birth

In the next week to ten days after birth the symbiotic relationship between you and your baby will continue. Gradually you will both adapt to each other and a rhythm will be established which will eventually become part of your family life.

Many changes take place at this time and you will find that for the first ten days at least you will need to be totally absorbed in this new adventure. You will need to have plenty of rest, to eat well and to more or less 'play it by ear' so you can discover how to attend to your baby's needs and find a natural rhythm. It helps if you take the line of least resistance, making your baby your first priority, sleeping when he sleeps and letting him be your guide. By following his needs you will find that harmony will prevail; by trying to impose a schedule of your own, life will become far more difficult for you.

How your body changes

After the birth your uterus will continue to contract each time your baby suckles and it will gradually become firmer and return to its pre-pregnant size and shape. This process takes between four and six weeks. At first these contractions may be uncomfortable and feel a little like menstrual cramps, but gradually these 'after pains' disappear and the contractions are painless and often pleasurable.

Bleeding will continue for a few weeks after the birth rather like a long period, but it will gradually lessen and cease. If you have had a perineal tear or epesiotomy and have had stitches, the wound will generally heal quite rapidly within the first fortnight. You can enhance your recovery by practising these simple exercises. Start as soon after the birth as you feel ready and build up slowly from 1 to 4 in your own time.

Exercise 1
Lie on your belly in bed or on the floor and tighten your pelvic floor muscles. Hold for a few seconds and then let go. Repeat ten to twenty times. This will help your perineum to return to normal and will facilitate healing.

Exercise 2
Do this after Exercise 1. Lie on your belly on the floor, arms by your sides. Lift up your head and your left leg. Hold for a few seconds, then relax. Then repeat lifting your right leg. Repeat ten to twenty times. This exercise strengthens the lower back and helps to firm the abdomen without strain.

Exercise 3
Do this after Exercises 1 and 2 and start after the seventh day. Lie on your belly on the floor. Tighten your buttocks, lift up your head and chest and rest your weight on your elbows, keeping your buttocks firm and your shoulders down away from your ears. Hold for a few seconds and then lie down and relax.

Repeat five times and be careful to keep your buttocks tight and not to hunch your shoulders. This exercise strengthens the lower back and helps to firm the abdomen.

Exercise 4
Roll over onto your back and draw your knees up to your chest, clasp your knees with your arms and breathe deeply. Hold for a few minutes. This relaxes and rests your lower back. Now let go of your knees, keeping them bent, and clasp your hands together. Reverse them palm outwards and stretch your arms up over your head onto the floor. Hold for a few minutes breathing deeply and then relax. Repeat a few times – this stretches the shoulders and relaxes the muscles which support your breasts.

During the early days after birth your body undergoes many hormonal changes as it returns to a non-pregnant state and begins to produce milk. You may well feel very emotional. You may have a 'post natal euphoria' and feel very high and elated for several days and even possibly weeks. It is also quite common to have a feeling of coming back to earth, a day of depression and weepiness. This usually coincides with the milk 'coming in' on the second or third day after the birth.

Preparing for breastfeeding and breastfeeding

During pregnancy your breasts prepare for producing milk and may become larger and more sensitive. The area surrounding the nipples may become darker in colour. It is not necessary to do anything special to prepare for feeding but it is a good idea to massage your breasts with some olive oil or almond oil after bathing and to wear a good supporting bra (preferably made of cotton). It is helpful to expose your breasts to fresh air and sunshine.

How your body makes milk
Your breasts, or mammary glands, are made up of fifteen to twenty-five segments called lobes, in which the milk is made. Each of these has its own duct system which converges on the nipple, widening out into little reservoirs called ampulae, just behind the nipple, which hold the milk. From here the ducts continue to the nipple opening. Around the ducts there are layers of fat which give the breasts their shape. Breast size differs in different women and small breasts produce milk just as well as large ones. The milk comes out of the little openings (or duct ends) in the nipple, like a fountain.

Towards the end of pregnancy you may notice a syrupy yellowish liquid leaking out of the nipples. This is called colostrum and is the first milk made by the breasts. It is richer

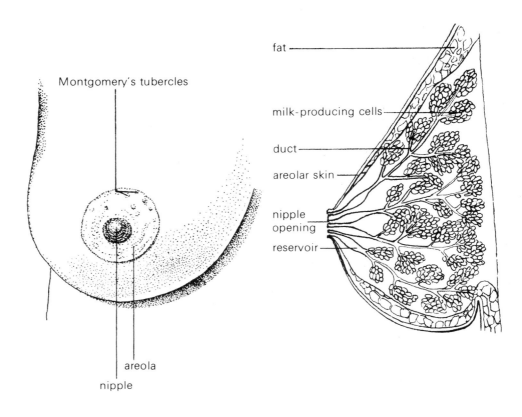

Montgomery's tubercles

fat

milk-producing cells

duct

areolar skin

nipple
opening

reservoir

areola

nipple

The breast

than mature breast milk in that it contains more protein and also antibodies which protect your baby from infection. It is the ideal first food for your baby for the first two days after birth and it does not need to be supplemented with water or any other food.

The earliest milk comes in two to three days after the birth and is still mixed with colostrum and looks rich and creamy. (By the tenth day it is much thinner and more watery.)

The milk usually comes in on the third day. You can expect to feel very emotional or even weepy. Your breasts can become very hard and full and much larger in size. This is known as engorgement and can be very uncomfortable, but after a few days the supply of milk will adjust itself to your baby's appetite and discomfort will pass. It is helpful to apply heat, such as frequent warm compresses, and to wear a good cotton maternity bra for support. Before feeding it may help to stand under a warm shower and massage the breasts from under the arms towards the nipple. Alternatively, try lying in a warm bath on your belly and let your breasts hang down in the water to ease the tension. You can express a little milk but it is best not to as this tends to stimulate the supply.

Breast milk is the ideal food for your baby, containing everything he or she needs, and it will suffice without any supplement for the first six to nine months at least. As your baby grows, sucking will increase, and this will stimulate or increase the milk production. It is an automatic supply-on-demand system.

It is important to be very comfortable and relaxed yourself while feeding your baby. Several positions are possible. Try sitting really upright, cross legged on the floor or in a comfortable chair, cradling your baby in your arms, with a cushion in your lap to support your arm and with your back well supported. Alternatively, try lying down sideways on a pile of cushions with your baby lying beside you in the crook of your arm. This is a very comfortable way to feed a baby in bed late at night.

When it is time for your baby to feed or when he begins to suck, you will feel a tingling sensation in the breasts as the milk begins to flow. This is called the 'let down reflex'. The milk that comes down in the first few minutes is the richest and most nutritious. After that it becomes more watery. Allowing your baby to feed as long as he wants to, perhaps falling asleep at the breast, provides him with warmth and comfort as well as food. Some babies suck for five to ten minutes and are full and satisfied, while others suck for hours. It takes a newborn twenty minutes to empty the breasts at first. Some babies latch onto the breast immediately and others need their interest aroused by squeezing a few drops of colostrum onto their lips or rubbing the nipple against the baby's cheek.

The best way to start the feeding is to allow your baby to be your guide. Feed baby whenever he or she is hungry and allow the baby to suckle comfortably as long as he wants to. Start with a different breast each time and make sure that the baby has the whole nipple, and not just the top part, in his or her mouth. The actual sucking is very powerful and will take a week or two to become comfortable and eventually highly enjoyable. If at first your nipples are painful then allow them to dry in the open air after feeding and rub a little almond oil into the areola and nipple, or alternatively, using a piece of cotton wool, dust them with a little slippery elm powder (available from health food stores). Don't wash too often; one bath a day is enough, and never use soap on your nipples as this removes the natural lubrication. Most women experience some soreness and discomfort when starting to breastfeed. Your baby may also experience difficulty with digestion of the rich milk at first. If your temperature rises or if your nipples become very painful or show signs of cracking, contact your midwife or doctor as soon as possible.

It is helpful to feed your baby like a gypsy – don't watch the clock and don't be surprised at the tremendous force of your baby's hunger. By taking the line of least resistance at first, a natural rhythm will evolve between your urge to feed and the complimentary desire of your baby. It is like a continuing circle and after you have overcome the possible initial difficulties, it will become a highly satisfying experience for you both.

How your baby changes

In the hours following the birth you will probably want to keep your baby very close to your body. It is not necessary to clothe the baby but he should be kept very warm, loosely wrapped in a soft shawl. Your body heat will help to keep your baby at the right temperature.

It is wise to put a soft nappy on the baby as he is likely to pass his first bowel movement some time in the twelve hours after the birth. This first bowel movement is known as meconium and is the substance that was in your baby's bowels in the womb. It is a sticky substance, dark green or blackish in colour. The colostrum or first milk which your breasts produce in the first two days helps to clear the baby's system of this meconium. When your baby begins to drink the normal breast milk around the third day, its bowel movement will gradually become yellow and sweet-smelling.

Jaundice

It is quite normal for some babies to appear slightly yellow, or jaundiced, around the second or third day after birth. This is caused by an excess of red blood cells in the baby's system. While in the womb, the baby needed these to handle its need for oxygen but after birth they are not needed and are broken down by the baby's body. A by-product of this breakdown is an excess of bilirubin which is deposited in the skin and is seen as a yellowish colouration and makes your baby look as if it has a suntan. The milk coming in will soon flush the baby's system clean. Sunshine helps to destroy the bilirubin so you could place the baby naked (with eyes shaded) in a warm spot in the sunlight for half-hour intervals. If the milk hasn't come in yet, try giving your baby a few drops of previously boiled water with an eyedropper or spoon at regular intervals.

The baby's cord

After the birth, the umbilical cord is usually clamped or tied and cut an inch or so away from the navel. It will begin to dry up immediately and will eventually fall off within the first ten days. You need to keep it dry and clean by folding the baby's nappies to that they don't rub against the cord. The cord can be cleaned with each nappy change using ten drops of Calendula mother tincture (homeopathic) in a little warm water. (This can also be used neat.)

Sleeping

Your baby will sleep for long periods in the early weeks, waking up only to feed. At first it is best to keep the baby very close to you, either on your body or beside you in bed, or else in a basket or crib at the side of the bed. Always place a newborn baby on his stomach to sleep so that any milk coming up will not choke him.

Carrying your baby

Babies love and need lots of close body contact, particularly at first when they have been used to being held all the time inside you. It is very helpful to use a baby-carrier – there are many available in the stores. These can be used within days after the birth by any member of the family and the baby can benefit from the warmth and security of being held while you do your shopping, go out for a walk or do any household tasks. This is often a very good way to calm a fretful baby.

Changing your baby

Your baby will urinate and empty his bowels frequently and you will need a good supply of nappies and simple baby clothes. You can change your baby before a feed or between breasts. It is best to avoid synthetic lotions, creams and powders and simply to wash your baby down with warm water and cotton wool, drying well afterwards in all the creases. Your baby should be dressed warmly at first. By the time they weigh eight pounds they can keep their body heat well and can be dressed more lightly. Their hands and feet should be just cool to the touch.

What to do when your baby cries

Babies usually cry when they are hungry – so that is probably the first thing to try. However, after some time you will learn to distinguish different cries for different needs. Trial and error is really the best way to find out – your baby may want to be held, rocked or to be changed, and sometimes just to express himself. It is impossible to spoil a newborn baby by giving him too much love, contact or attention and it doesn't help to allow a small baby to 'cry it out'. However, when faced with a baby that seems inconsolable, the best you can do is try every way to comfort him or pass him on to someone else to try. Most babies have a time of day in which they tend to be rather fretful and, of course, if you are stressed or anxious yourself you are likely to pass these feelings on to your baby. Generally babies that are held and breastfed on demand are likely to be perfectly contented and peaceful most of the time. However, young babies often experience some difficulties at first with digestion. If this is the case, try 'burping' the baby after feeding by holding him over your shoulder and patting his back, or else lay him on his belly on your lap and stroke his back. Sometimes massaging his belly gently can be helpful. It may take you a few weeks to know your baby and how best to help him when he cries. No one can know a baby as well as his own mother.

Kalongo, a Kikiyu chief of East Africa, spoke these words (taken from *Touching* by Ashley Montague) when he was eighty years of age:

My early years are connected in my mind with my mother. At first she was always there; I can remember the comforting feel of her body as she carried me on her back and the smell of her skin in the hot sun. Everything came from her. When I was hungry or thirsty she would swing me round to where I could reach her full breasts; now when I shut my eyes I feel again with gratitude the sense of well-being that I had when I buried my head in their softness and drank the sweet milk that they gave. At night when there was no sun to warm me, her arms, her body, took its place; and as I grew older and more interested in other things, from my safe place on her back I could watch without fear as I wanted and when sleep overcame me I had only to close my eyes.

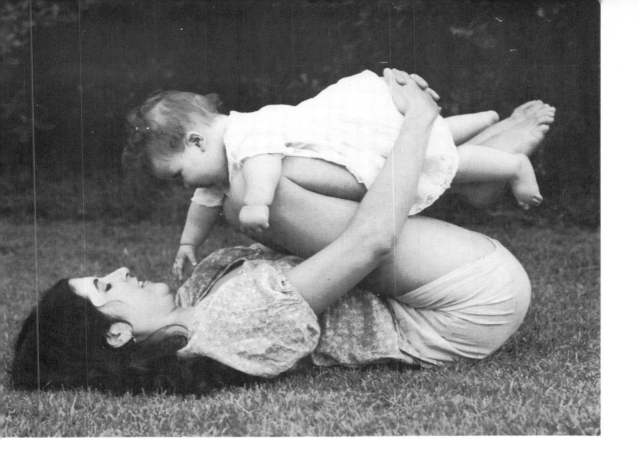

Getting back to normal

After several months you may want and need to do some exercises that would hasten the return of your figure to normal. The following positional exercises are suggested to do just that. They can be done while your child is asleep, probably the most convenient time is when he or she is taking an afternoon nap, or they can be done, weather permitting, with your baby outdoors, as shown in the photographs.

Above: Lying on back flexing hips and knees

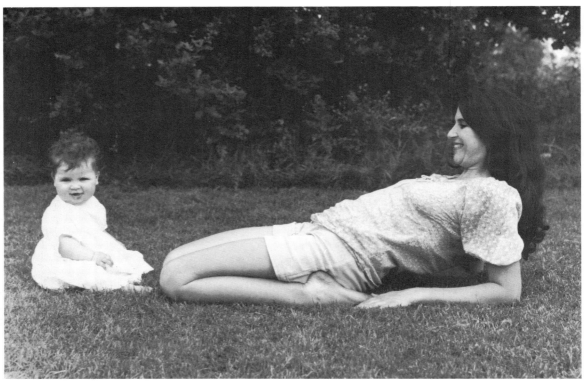
Sitting between feet and lying back on elbows

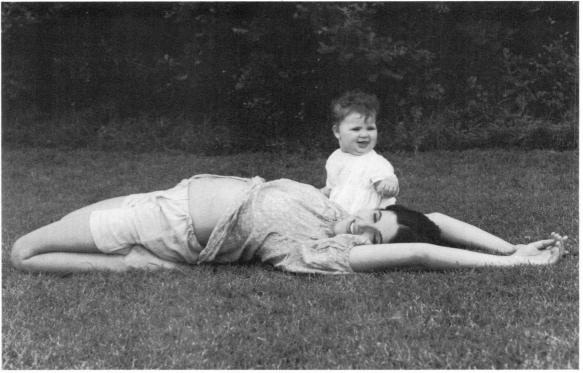
Sitting between feet and lying back with arms overhead

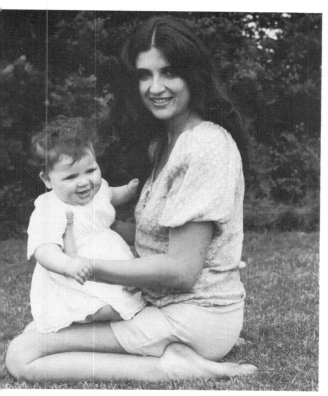

Sitting between feet

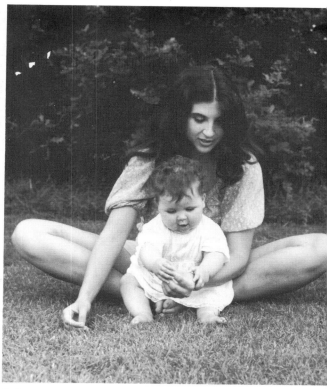

Tailor position

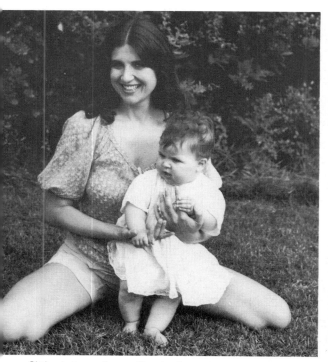

Sitting between feet and leaning forward

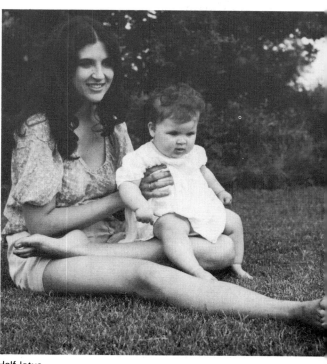

Half-lotus

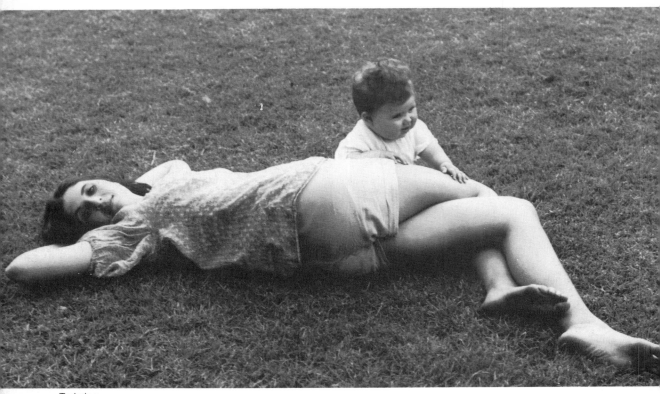

Twisting

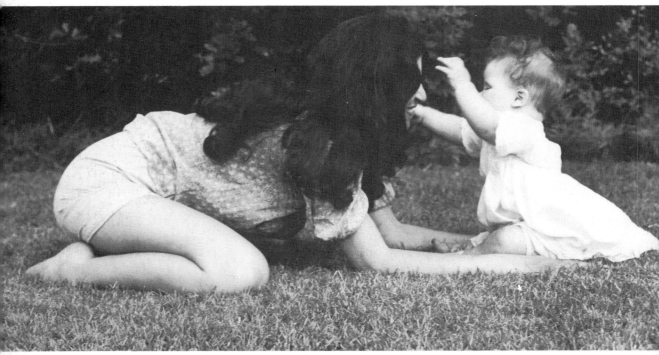

Sitting on heels with knees spread apart

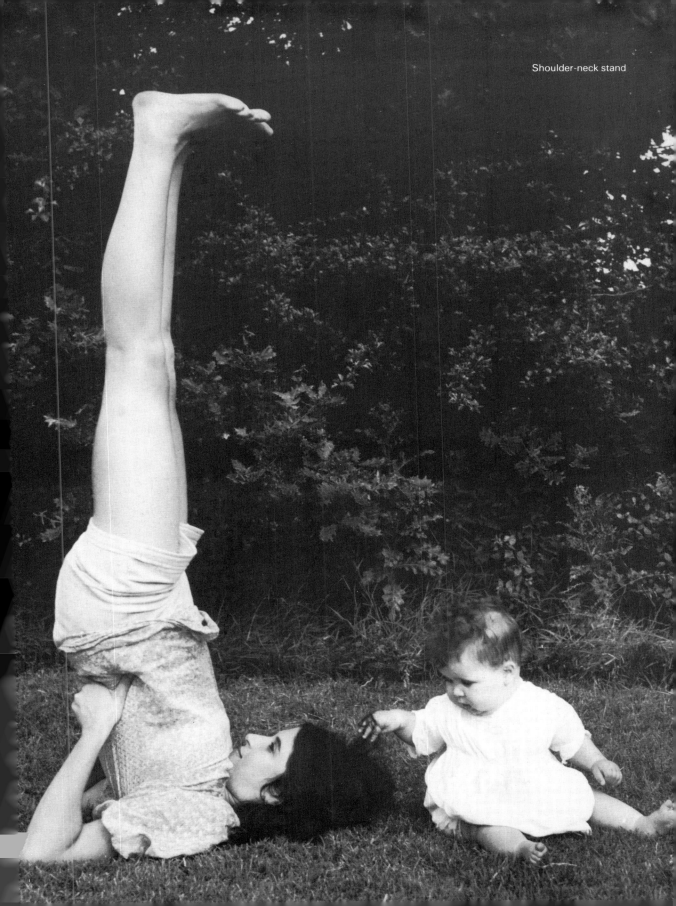

Shoulder-neck stand

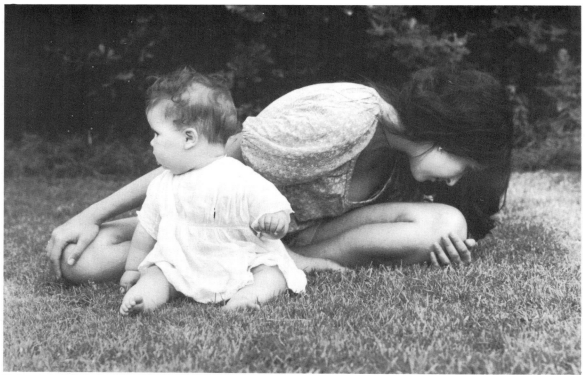

Sitting easy and bending to knee

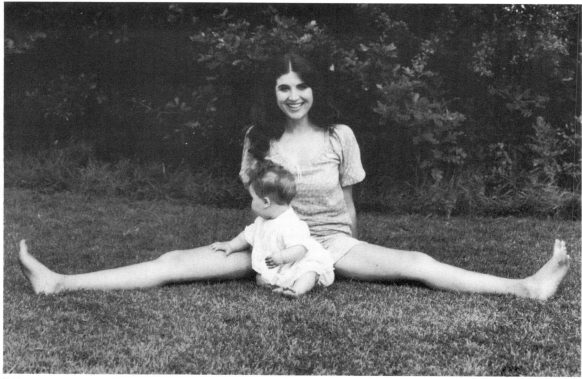

Sitting with knees straight and spread apart

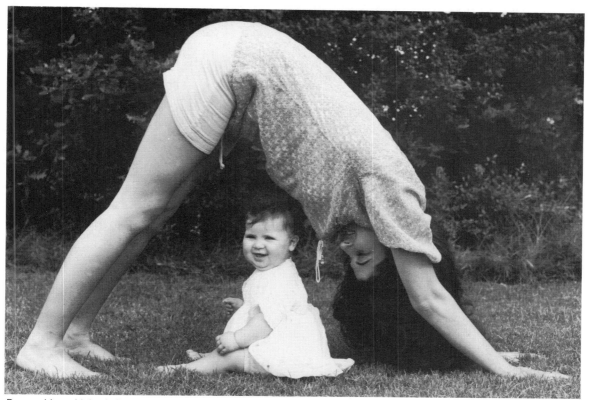
Dog position with heels flat on ground

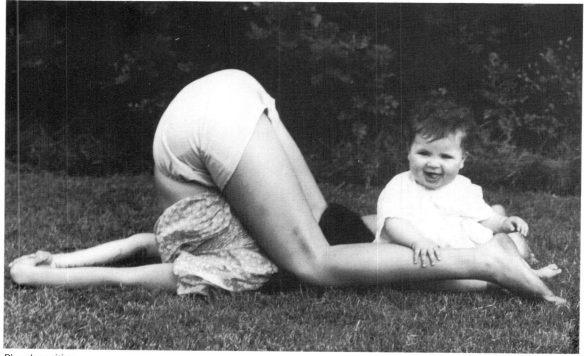
Plough position

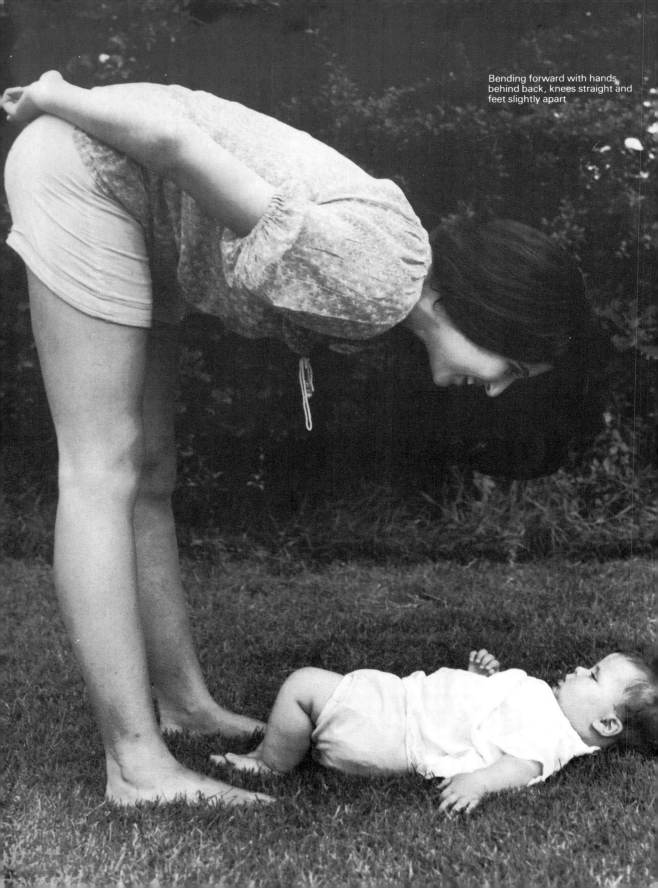

Bending forward with hands
behind back, knees straight and
feet slightly apart

Index